WHAT EVERY MAN NEEDS TO KNOW

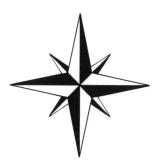

How to Master Faith, Family, Fitness and Finances

TODD ISBERNER

This book is written with gratitude to the mentors God surrounded me with in the very beginning: Doug, Rich, Mike, and Paul. And to my band of brothers of the last 30 years, thank you for the privilege of walking it out with each of you in the real world.

Editor: Ronald Olson (ron@ronaldolson.com)

Cover and Interior Design: Kayla J Nelson (kayla.j.nelson@outlook.com)

FACEBOOK: WHAT EVERY MAN NEEDS TO KNOW

www.facebook.com/todd.isberner

WEBSITE: www.toddisberner.com
todd@toddisberner.com
www.whateverymanneedsto know.com

ISBN-13: 978-0-578-42941-0

TABLE OF CONTENTS

WHAT EVERY MAN NEEDS TO KNOW

How to Master Faith, Family,
Fitness and Finances

INTRODUCTION

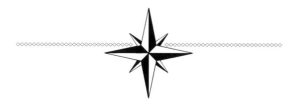

"Act like a man!"

Ever hear that one? It was a line used by parents with little boys who usually were whining about something they didn't like.

So do you act like a man? Or are you not completely sure what that even means?

You have no doubt heard the fable about an eagle that thought he was a chicken. When the eagle was very small he fell from his nest and a chicken farmer rescued him. He put the eagle in with all of his chickens. So the eagle grew up doing what chickens do, strutting around clucking, scratching and pecking at the ground and acting like a chicken.

It wasn't until a naturalist came by and noticed the farmer had an eagle acting like a chicken. After convincing the farmer that this was an eagle who could soar above the heights, he set out to prove his point.

He raised the eagle up on his arm and told it to fly, but it dropped back down to the ground and started pecking. Then he took the eagle to the top of the barn and told it to fly. But again, it fluttered back down to the ground and continued strutting and clucking.

Finally, the naturalist took the eagle to the top of a mountain, no longer in sight of the chicken coops, the barn and the farm. He told the eagle to stretch out its wings and fly. This time the eagle stared skyward into the bright sun, straightened its large body and stretched its massive wings. His wings moved, slowly at first, then surely and powerfully. With the mighty screech of an eagle he flew!

I think you get the point. *Sometimes, all we know how to be is that which has been modeled for us or imposed upon us.*

Are you an eagle acting like a chicken? Or a man living out his fullness of what it really means to act like a man?

So what exactly is a man and how can he reestablish his core beliefs about who he is and how he can function in his peak *manness*?

And why do we even need to ask?

Because in today's world, although there are noticeable external differences between men and women, the core internal makeup of a what a man is has been severely marred. If he in any way takes on a traditional approach to living out his life as a man, then expressing his distinctly male characteristics through his beliefs, thoughts, feelings and actions, will often be challenged by the world around him.

And yet, God wired into each man's heart some core desires that if not fulfilled, can lead to confusion, ineptness in his role and fear that can cripple his potential.

In John Eldridge's classic book, *Wild at Heart*, he elaborates on what these core desires are and what can happen if you live them out.

1. A battle to fight: for his life, his marriage, his dreams, his integrity.
2. An adventure to live: to take risks, to explore, to break free.
3. A beauty to rescue: to live out his role as hero, provider, protector.

God has made you with a purpose and role that perfectly suits your internal desires. But if you are not free to pursue them, and instead deny or hide from them, you can never experience the fullness of what it means to be a man!

The reality is that your manhood is being reshaped today by a new set of expectations that require you to align with the externally-imposed cultural and politically correct standards. In this politically correct cultural norm, today's man is supposed to conform to the image of a genderless human who is perfectly the same as all other humans.

This is of course utter nonsense!

The very fact that there are physiological differences in the human body between a man and a woman should tell us that our God-created differences should be celebrated. The differences in the makeup of a man versus a woman naturally result in a difference in the way each gender functions.

We function differently because we are different! There will be differences in what we believe about ourselves and in the way we think, feel and act.

The outcome of those differences results in a distinction of roles as well. And that can be a very good thing in that it contributes to a balance of life that equalizes the value of each gender.

With that in mind, I'm going to lay out four foundational pillars in life that every man needs to stand on every day. Developing routines and disciplines within these four areas of life determine how well a man can function within his role as a protector, provider and leader.

The four FOUNDATIONAL areas of life that affect every man, every day are:

1. FAITH
The internal core of what aligns a man with his creator to become who he is designed to be, and live out his purpose.

2. FAMILY
The central place of community that shapes a society.

3. FITNESS
The physical, mental and spiritual strength that gives the stamina and perseverance it takes to fulfill a man's potential.

4. FINANCES
The currency that fuels the freedom to provide for those in a man's care and contribute to the needs of others.

Learning to master these four foundational areas that encompass your life will give you freedom to live out your purpose and fulfill your role.

The word master can have multiple meanings and has been popularized to the point of losing its impact. Jim, a friend of mine who ran my business, would often mimic Darth Vader's voice from Star Wars when asking me (tongue in cheek), *"Master, what is thy bidding?"*

That's not necessarily what we're referring to here. Although, putting it into another context, we are going to learn what our ultimate Master/Teacher/Lord has for us in these four areas of life. (More about that in the next section.)

But for our purposes here, we're going to use master as an action verb.

To master is to learn the skills needed to become proficient in overcoming the fears and the challenges in these four key areas of life.

And what's the point in mastering your faith, family, fitness and finances? Is it just for the sake of becoming a better you? Will it cause you to become even more self-absorbed, trying to reach the pinnacle of all you can be? Perhaps. But only if you are too short-sighted to see the bigger picture.

It's not just about you, and you don't want it that way anyhow. Nobody wants to be selfish and no one wants to be around someone who is. But if the outcome of mastering these areas can cause me to be better equipped to help others, then I can avoid self-centered motives.

Any one of these areas can consume the majority of your time and attention. And to the degree that you have not learned to master them, you will inevitably experience a compounding effect of problems that create stress, chaos and unavoidable, hurtful consequences for you and those around you.

For example, maybe you're not really sure the whole **faith** thing is relevant. God is **out there** somewhere, and you're slugging it out here on planet earth, so why think He would be involved in the details of your everyday life? Or you just don't know enough about the whole subject and don't want to take the time to learn.

Maybe you've had faith at one point in your life, but God seems to have ignored you or let you down or worse yet, punished you. So why bother? This puts you on shaky ground, leaving you without a firm belief that God loves you and wants good for you. As a result, nothing else can really come together the way you hope it could.

Perhaps you've struggled with your **family relationships** and no matter how hard you try, it seems like there is nothing you can do to fix it. Or maybe you're aware that things could be better, but your work is so all consuming that you think you have to put making a living first.

And now, you're suffering the effects of family members who judge you, don't trust you, and feel ignored, unloved and uncared for. Worse yet, you may already have crossed over the line and have such brokenness in the relationship that you are convinced it's too late and things are over.

Your **health and fitness** is something you know needs more attention, but you don't have the time or the energy to make the effort or even have the want-to. You know that if you lost some weight, reshaped your physique, had more stamina and drive, everything else in life would feel the positive effects. But you simply don't have the discipline, the know-how or the right motivation to make it a priority.

Your health is at risk and maybe you are already experiencing the decline in the way your body should perform. You don't want it that way, but feel almost helpless in changing it, to the point that you can't even imagine what it would be like to function at your peak performance.

When it comes to **finances**, are you so in control that you feel invincible? Or are you so out of control that you feel enslaved? Have you measured success, or lack of it, by how much you earn, how much you owe or how much or little is in your bank account? Ever get in so deep you've been on the verge of bankruptcy, or already declared it?

Has your financial position kept you up at night, and like a computer program always running in the background, money is constantly on your mind? Or maybe things are just "okay," and while you're "getting by," it never seems like you can really get ahead with enough reserve to take the pressure off.

Do you want to give yourself the best shot at reversing things so you can overcome what is causing you pain and holding you back? Want to get to the place where you can truly maximize your potential and start celebrating who you are as a confident, successful man, capable of leading others?

Then take the first step and come clean. Have an open and honest conversation with yourself. Acknowledge where you're struggling so you can go into attack mode and learn to master it.

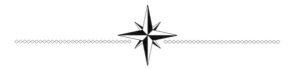

❏ Take a moment right now and think about which of these four foundational areas of life are already causing pain for you. Write it down.

❏ What are the consequences of not having it under control?

❏ Besides you, who else is being affected by it?

❏ How would life look differently if this area was mastered?

You may already have one or more of these four areas somewhat mastered. But thinking that you don't need to improve will short-circuit your growth. EVERY man has opportunity to learn more and become more proficient in each one of these areas. Doing so earns you the expertise to master all four of these crucial areas of life and gives you the confidence to be successful and to serve others.

Now, I don't particularly care for How-To books. Most men don't. We don't like to be told how to do things. We like to figure things out on our own. We like our independence and have an image of ourselves as mavericks able to blaze our own trail. The only problem is that even if we know where we want to end up, we don't always know how to get there. How many times while driving somewhere have you stubbornly refused directions because you thought you knew the way, but you ended up lost.

Real men ask for help when they need it!

A number of years ago, I finally came to the realization that I could use some help when it came to mastering things that I didn't have expertise in. It wasn't because I didn't want to tackle these areas. It's just that I didn't have the experience to qualify me to know how to master these areas of life.

Let's face it, if we are willing to set our egos aside, show some transparent vulnerability and ask for help, we put ourselves in a position to learn, grow, succeed and lead.

Without some basic instructions in these four key areas of life, we can easily get confused, off track, unproductive and ineffective. The decisions you make and the actions you take will cause outcomes that will either make or break you.

So consider this book more of a guide to help you learn and successfully implement the skills needed to overcome the challenges you face in each of these areas.

Vince Lombardi, one of the greatest football coaches of all time started every season the same way. On the practice field facing his eager team of players, he would start the first practice by saying, "Gentlemen, this is a football."

Then, practice after practice, he ran his players through the most elementary drills of catching, throwing, blocking and tackling. It was all about knowing the basic fundamentals and practicing them over and over until they were imbedded within his players.

And as the saying goes, "It's not, practice makes perfect, but practice makes permanent!"

> We need to make permanent those practices that are wise, disciplined and consistent, so we can master our faith, family, fitness and finances. You are meant to succeed and lead. But to do so requires that you keep learning, growing and most importantly, doing.

This book is laid out in the form of a handbook. I was going to call it a workbook, but the truth is, few men want to feel like they are adding more work to their day.

So as a handbook, it is full of insights, instructions and exercises. You can use it as a training manual, a journal, a reference guide, a personalized map for what you plan on doing and how. Interact with the questions in each area.

Underline, highlight, take notes and write down action plans. Use the references. Commit to completing each section with no shortcuts. Measure your progress and it will help you stay motivated.

Take each section seriously, slowly and with the commitment to master it. These four areas have to be learned to be earned, and learning is locked in by the doing.

So let's get to it.

FAITH

✝

OXFORD DICTIONARY DEFINITION:

1. complete trust or confidence in someone or something.
2. strong belief and trust in and loyalty to God or in the doctrines of a religion, based on spiritual apprehension rather than proof.

BIBLE DEFINITION:

"Now faith is the substance of things hoped for, the evidence of things not seen."
Hebrews 11:1 (KJV)

1

Know Your Starting Point.

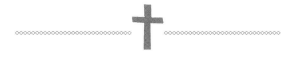

To some, this first area of life would be a no-brainer. Of course you need faith, and you need to be strong in faith for everything else to line up in the way in which it was designed.

It would seem reasonable that if there is a God who made you, He must have had a reason or a purpose for wanting you here. And with a purpose comes a plan that was designed specifically for you. So then, the more you get to know God, the more you will understand His purpose and plan for your life. Then within your role as a man, you will be able to function best in all areas of life.

I'm writing this book on a computer. I didn't make the computer so I can't possibly understand all the technical intricacies that makes this computer function the way it does. At the same time, I have the opportunity to continually learn how to best use this computer. The manufacturer has already provided all kinds of helps built within the software. All I need to do is take the time to search, learn and apply.

But I would never be so arrogant as to think that just because I can do some basic functions on my computer that it somehow makes me an expert. No, I depend on the manufacturer's expertise when I want to use all the functions that make this computer perform at its best.

So it is with knowing how to function at your best as a man. The God who designed you knows how He "wired" you, and wants you to learn from Him and depend on Him.

I had a framed print hanging on a wall that was a constant reminder to me.

It says:

> *There are two foundational truths.*
> *1. There is a God.*
> *2. You are not Him.*

With that in mind, let's go to the starting point, "In the beginning God...."

This is the classic, well-known, first line of the Bible in Genesis chapter 1, and it states an all important truth: there is a God and it all starts with Him. He is the creator of all things seen and unseen. He is your creator and He made you in His image. He made you for a reason and has a purpose and plan for your life.

If you're not sure about any of that, then it's not likely you know Him or have a relationship with Him. You may know something about Him, but that's a whole lot different than actually knowing Him personally. And if you don't know Him, how will you know who you are meant to be and what your purpose in life is?

There really is no point in trying to live out your full potential as a man if you are not in an intimate relationship with the God who made you. He knows you and you need to know Him.

The Bible says that God thought about you even before He laid out the foundations of this earth. And before you were born, He numbered all your days and laid out every moment of every single day. Then He knit you together in your mother's womb, creating you to be His masterpiece (Ephesians 2:10, Psalm 139:13).

He knows everything about you. He knows your thoughts and the words on your lips even before you speak them, your hopes and dreams, your future victories and failures. There is nothing hidden from Him and nowhere you can go that puts you out of His presence and awareness (Psalm 139).

The truth is, He made you because He loves you and wants you to know Him.

So do you? Do you know about Him, or do you really know Him, personally? And if not, why?

Yet, no matter how badly you want to know Him or how hard you try, it's simply not possible on your own. The problem is, you are a sinner. Me too.

And sin puts us at a distance from God. It separates us simply because God is Holy (perfect and sinless) and He cannot commingle with sin. It's not even within His nature to be able to sin. God is love and sin is rooted in hate, pride and evil.

"All men have sinned and fall short of the glory of God." Romans 3:23 (NASB)

And that describes the human condition, your condition, unless your sin has been removed and your sinful nature put down.

In the beginning of the creation of man, God set up the rules (out of love and protection for us). He also set up the consequences for living under the control of the sinful nature and He judges the guilty.

The sentence? Death penalty. Meaning eternal death, permanent separation from the God who made you and loves you.

Pretty depressing, huh?

But here's the really incredibly great news; God loves you too much to let you be separated from Him. So He Himself did something about it since He knew you couldn't.

God became a man 2,000 years go in the form of Jesus the Christ. And He proved His divine nature by all the miracles He did like raising the dead, healing the blind, the lame, the deaf, multiplying loaves and fishes, walking on water, even changing water into wine! Who does that?

Jesus did. Because he was the God-man who lived in a human body so he could experience everything you do in exactly the same way. With one exception that is. Jesus never sinned! (Even though he was fully human, like you.)

And because He loved you so much, He offered Himself as a perfect, sinless sacrifice on your behalf. He took upon Himself your death sentence so you could be forgiven and set free!

He was put to death by a torturous, horrific crucifixion and buried in a tomb.

But then after three days, the ultimate miracle took place – He took on life again! He literally rose from the dead!

Jesus conquered death and overcame the power of sin and its consequences. He did that for you because He loves you and wants you to spend eternity in Heaven.

Jesus has been given all authority in Heaven and on earth. He rules over everything and has earned the right to judge everyone. And because He has substituted His life for yours, He now has a claim on your life.

So here's what it comes down to; your FAITH in Jesus and what He did for you.

It's your admission that you are a sinner and need His grace, forgiveness and salvation. That alone is what gives you access to God in an intimate relationship with Him now and forever.

However, it's one thing to just believe it and a whole other thing to act on it.

Acting on it means you invite the Spirit of Jesus to literally come inside of you to live His life through you. (Yes, you will be indwelt by His Spirit.)

"Behold I stand at the door and knock (the door of your heart), if anyone hears my voice and opens the door, I will come into him and dine with him." Revelation 3:20 (NASB)

When you make your confession of faith and invite His Spirit to come live inside of you, you are agreeing to surrender your own will to His will, and making a commitment to follow Him all the days of your life.

And He promises He will be with you always and will never leave you nor forsake you (Matthew 28:20, Hebrews 13:5).

Have you done that? Have you asked Jesus to come into your heart and take control of your life? If not, do it right now.

Talk to God in your own words, and if you're not sure what to say, let this prompt you.

"Lord Jesus, I need You. I confess I have sinned and lived my own life apart from You. I believe You love me and gave Yourself on my behalf so I could be forgiven and cleansed and set free. I surrender all of my life to You Lord, and ask that You come live inside me and make me the man You want me to be. I give You all my praise for who You are and what You've done. I love You Lord. I thank You Lord. I am Yours, Lord!"

This is incredibly good news for you because the Bible says, *"What happiness for those whose guilt has been forgiven. What joys when sins are covered over. What relief for those who have confessed their sins and God has cleared their record."* Psalm 32:1-2 (TLB)

God's Word says that you are now ready to live out His purpose for you because, *"You are God's masterpiece, a new creation in Christ Jesus, so that you can do the good things He already prepared in advance for you to do"* (Ephesians 2:10).

Once your life is surrendered to Jesus, you will have His Spirit living inside of you, empowering you through every moment of every day. *"[You] can do all things through Christ who gives you strength"* (Philippians 4:13).

You will experience *"His mighty power at work within you, to accomplish infinitely more than you would ever dare to ask or hope for"* (Ephesians 3:20). And you will be filled with a passion to share this life-changing good news with others.

MY OWN STORY OF FAITH.

Staring through the stained-glass window of the chapel, I thought I heard God calling me to the priesthood. I was in the fourth grade and loved serving mass as an altar boy. It made me feel close to God.

But that "calling" quickly faded when I turned 15 and discovered girls, athletics and parties. The innocence of my childhood years began to disappear the moment I started making bad decisions. That led me down a path that took me away from God.

For the following ten years, I put my faith on hold and lived more like a rebel without a cause. It all caught up with me when I was 25, going through an unwanted divorce as a father of a five-year-old daughter. I wasn't much of a husband and had a huge ego that convinced me I was in control of my life.

My neighbors had been talking to me about Jesus and the Bible and I laughed it off as a "crutch" for weak people. But when it all came crashing down, I found myself face down, begging God for help.

I met with their pastor who listened to my side of the story, and rather than sympathize, he lovingly said, "Do you realize this whole thing is your fault?"

My fault? How could this be?

He told me I needed to get right with God by owning up to the decisions that led me away from Him. He showed me passages from God's Word that helped me see how I was responsible for the sin and chaos in my life. I needed God's forgiveness and could freely receive His love because of what Jesus did for me on the cross.

It seemed too easy, but I surrendered, opened up my heart and asked Jesus to come live inside me. It shook me to the core.

Actually, it was His Spirit that shook me as I literally wept with sorrow and then joy over the discovery of God's amazing grace and love for me.

From that moment on, everything changed. My thinking, my attitudes, my behavior. Everything about me was being transformed by a power within me that I had never known. I had purpose and meaning!

Although I had a new outlook on life, life didn't get easier. But with a new found faith and guidance from God's Word and Spirit, handling the challenges of life got a lot easier.

What about you?

Have you come to the place in life where you have experienced God's forgiveness, love and presence within you? If not, I encourage you – no I implore you –open up your heart and by faith, receive the new life He has for you, and discover the real purpose and meaning to your life.

❏ If you made a decision to commit or renew your life to Christ, write in your owns words your declaration of commitment to Jesus, and date it.

❏ Write down who you're going to tell about it and when.

Now that you have established, or reestablished your starting point, where do you go from here?

2

Set your FAITH growing goals.

✝

"Aim at nothing and you will hit it every time."

Maybe it sounds a bit strange to set goals when it comes to spiritual matters. But unless there is intentional planning and doing, your faith will become ineffective.

Shortly after I gave my life to the Lord Jesus at age 25, I realized I needed to work daily on growing my faith. I knew God wanted to transform me into someone who looked and acted more like Jesus. But I also knew that I couldn't just sit back unengaged and somehow, mystically become a new person in Christ. I had already been setting goals in other areas of my life and figured setting faith goals needed to take top priority.

NOTE: Before setting goals, I'm going to suggest that if you haven't already done so, first make certain you have an overarching mission statement for your life.

All that really amounts to is answering the question, "What on earth am I here for?" Knowing your purpose motivates you to live it out with intention. And it prepares you for eternity.

» **Check out Rick Warren's daily plan for a Purpose Driven life here:** www.purposedriven.com/day1/
This is a daily video series by Rick Warren that gives you a great starting place in understanding why God made you and what your purpose is all about.

Take some time now and answer these questions. Then, based on your answers, summarize them in your own personal mission statement.

❏ Why am I alive?

❏ Why do I think God put me here?

❏ Does my life matter? How do I know?

☐ What's His purpose for me?

☐ Am I living it out? If not, what is preventing me from fulfilling my purpose?

☐ What drives my life? Do I want or need that to change?

☐ Up to this point in my life, what am I doing that brings me the greatest satisfaction in knowing I'm living out my purpose?

☐ Write out *My Mission Statement*.

Once you have the purpose for your life solidly anchored in your heart and soul, then move into a goal-setting mode. This will help you be more intentional about growing your faith and living out your purpose for being here.

When I first surrendered my life to the Lord, I went to the Bible to see if I could find a starting place for setting goals to grow my faith.

There is a letter in the Bible written by the Apostle Peter who wanted to instruct the new believers (and us) on how to grow in our knowledge of God, which would result in living an effective life as a follower of Jesus.

He reassured us that God has given us His "precious promises" that enable us to share in His divine nature. And as we participate in God's nature, we can practice on a daily basis the behaviors that cause us to grow.

To paraphrase 2 Peter 1:3-10:
By his divine power, God has given us everything we need for living a godly life. For this very reason, make every effort to add to your faith moral excellence; and moral excellence with knowledge, and knowledge with self-control, and self-control with patient endurance, and patient endurance with godliness, and godliness with brotherly affection, and brotherly affection with love for everyone. ***The more you grow like this, the more productive and useful you will be in your knowledge of our Lord Jesus Christ. Do these things and you will never fall away.***

Quite the list, huh?

At first it can seem a bit overwhelming and unrealistic, and rightfully so if you try it in your own strength. But remember, you have the Holy Spirit of Jesus living in you and can rely on His strength and power.

So let's break it down. You want to set goals that grow your faith and can be practiced on a daily basis. The evidence of achieving those goals will be seen in your core values and the lifestyle behaviors found in 2 Peter 1:3-10.

In other words, your life will start looking more like the life of Jesus.

When it comes to setting faith-growing goals, it's important to keep in mind that they are not the end all of your faith journey. Rather, they are stepping stones that guide you and keep you moving in the right direction as you live out your Christian life. It's much like adapting a core values lifestyle strategy as you work on your goals.

So the question is, what faith goals can you create that can be implemented on a daily basis within the current circumstances of your life?

You probably already know that when setting goals, it is always more powerful to write them out. They need to be specific and they need to be achievable.

While everyone's individual goals and plans for accomplishing them will be uniquely designed, here is an example of what it could look like. This is some of what I outlined for my own faith goals at the beginning of my journey.

1. As soon as I get out of bed, get on my knees and acknowledge Jesus as Lord and Savior and name every area of my life I am surrendering back to Him.

2. Commit to a Quiet Time for devotions and prayer for at least 15 minutes every day, first thing in the morning. (More details about this in the next section.)

3. Use a daily scripture reading plan and read through the Bible in a year.

4. Once per week, write down in a journal at least one page of insights and how I will apply what God is showing me.

5. Memorize at least one scripture per week.

6. Every day pray for the faith, growth and spiritual protection for my children, family and those who God has entrusted to me.

7. Attend a Bible-believing church every Sunday.

8. Join a weekly men's Bible study and commit to attending and to being held accountable in my faith walk.

9. Share the gospel with someone at least once per month.

10. Every day, be intentional in finding at least one person to encourage and serve.

While this might be a suggested starting place, you may have something completely different in mind in terms of goals that will help you grow your faith. But if it isn't a deliberate and intentional pursuit, you will stagnate and not grow.

☐ So before going further, take some time right now (or schedule a time later), to think about and pray through your goals. Write them down. Put them in your smartphone. Look at them every day and measure your progress every week.

We never grow closer to God when we just live life. It takes deliberate pursuit and attentiveness." - Francis Chan

3

Practice Quiet Times
for Daily Devotions.

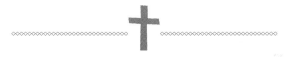

Quiet time simply means taking a brief period of time to quiet oneself from all distractions and spend it reading God's Word, meditating on what He says and talking it over with Him. I, along with many others, refer to this daily practice as a Quiet Time. Some call it devotions, God time, etc., and you can call it anything you want as a way of describing a designated time you will spend meeting with God.

Just as sleep is required for the body to regenerate on a daily basis, so is a daily quiet time needed to rejuvenate the spirit.

Being sleep-deprived can cause severe and permanent physical and mental problems. It's probably why sleep deprivation has been used as a torture technique when looking to break down a captive.

Depriving our spirit time to connect intimately with God can also lead to all kinds of problems. We can become severely handicapped in living out a vibrant, spiritually strong and intimate relationship with God. Without daily quiet time, intentionally planned out, we can become vulnerable to the deceptions of our enemy, the devil.

There is a devil (called Lucifer or Satan), and he rules and directs armies of demonic powers. There is an invisible world all around you, whether you believe it or not. And because these demonic forces are at war with God and His angelic beings, you are caught up in it, because YOU are the target.

The devil's goal is to discredit and disprove God. He is trying to prove a point that with his influence, little finite human beings like you will reject the invisible Creator God, and that you will instead choose to be your own god.

With you being your own god, you get to:
• make decisions for yourself based on your own preferences.
• exercise your "right" to live the way you want to.
• control everything in your life the way you want it to be, regardless of what anyone else thinks or wants, including the Creator God.
• maintain this self-ruling position as god over your own life, thinking it will make you happy, prosperous and successful in all things.

Tell me that lie wasn't at work within you before you fully surrendered to God?

Jesus called Satan the father of lies. So because you are the devil's target, you need to be all the more anchored in your faith by immersing yourself in God and His truth.

That's the benefit of spending intimate time everyday with the God who made you, loves you and wants you to know Him. As a result, you WILL know the truth, and Jesus promised that the truth WILL set you free.

So let's dig into some basics for having a Quiet Time.

1. First, make a commitment to have a Quiet Time every day.

Determine the value it has in your life. View it equally as important as food for your body or the oxygen you need to breathe.

❏ Write out your commitment. Sign and date it.

2. Prioritize your Quiet Time.

This really has to be your first and most important activity of your day. It's likely that every day you have to decide which things you're going to do that have the highest priority. If you make a list of things to do, put this as number 1!

3. Choose a place and schedule a time daily to have your Quiet Time.

For most people, first thing in the morning seems to work well. It helps set the day in the right direction with the determination to follow the Lord's lead. Select a comfortable spot that keeps you free from distractions. I have a favorite chair by the window. But yours could be something entirely different that best suits your needs. I've heard of everything from having it in the car in the parking lot outside work, to a busy mom with little kids retreating to a closet. Whatever location you select, view it as a sanctuary where you can meet one-on-one with God.

4. Read God's Word.

There are so many great Bible reading plans with a variety of ways to go through the Scriptures. Almost every year since I surrendered my life to Christ, I make it a goal to read through the Bible in a year. It has been the number one way for me to gain God's perspective on who He is and how He relates to us.

»Two very popular Bible reading apps are:
YouVersion (www.youversion.com), and **Read Scripture** (www. readscripture.org).

Check them out or find something else that helps you move deeper into God's Word with consistency. (You might also want to add to this a devotional reading of some kind like My Utmost for His Highest or Jesus Calling.)

5. Use a journal to record your thoughts and insights.

This does not have to be a lengthy nor complicated process. As you read or when you've finished reading a section of Scripture, simply write down a few words, phrases or sentences that express your insights. Make it personal and make it applicable.

6. Pray.

This is not some kind of formal, lengthy, religious ritual. Rather it is simply a conversation, in your own words, talking with God about the insights He shared with you. You will want to praise Him for who He is, thank Him for what He's done, and like a child with his father, ask Him for what you (or others) need.

7. Make it count.

Find the one thing from your time spent with God that you will take with you throughout the day. Make it something you can apply to your everyday life as a tangible action item.

Just to illustrate a bit, here's an example of how I did a Quiet Time.

• 6:30am - Brought my coffee and Bible to favorite chair near the window.

• 6:30-6:45 - Read a section of the Bible (Hebrews chapter 5) from a one year reading plan.

• 6:45-6:55 - Selected one thing that stood out most and decided how I can apply it. (Verse 2: we are priests or mediators who are to help the wayward while being aware of our own weaknesses. Call the person God put on my heart and encourage him today.)

• 6:55-7:00 - Talked with God about it, and then gave Him thanks and praise for who He is and what He has done. Finished with special requests, mostly on behalf of others.

Obviously this is just a simple sample. I'm not that rigid or disciplined to make this so exact that I lose out on the flexibility and freedom God gives when it comes to spending time with Him. There are times where I just sit and think and pray for 10 minutes – or for an hour.

But the bottom line is to have a consistent, daily time to spend with God. It will rest and refresh your soul. *"Come away with me. Let us go alone to a quiet place and rest for awhile"* (Mark 6:31).

4

Walk it Out.

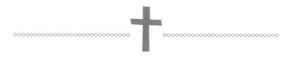

Maybe you've observed in your own life or heard it said of someone that they talk a good game, but don't live it out. Let's face it, authentic Christianity is proved by the way it is lived out in our everyday lives. But, too often it is a lot easier to just talk about God and the Christian life than it is to actually live it.

We have such an abundance of spiritual helps and resources through books, apps, podcasts and conferences. You can choose any Bible translation you want and go to any church of your preferred flavor. With all that's available to pack our heads full of all the knowledge we could ever need, if we're not careful we could end up *ever learning, but never doing.*

In the Bible, the book of James says it pretty directly. *"Do not merely listen to God's word. But do what it says. Otherwise you are only fooling yourselves. For if you listen to the word and don't do it, it is like glancing at your face in the mirror. You see yourself, walk away, and forget what you look like"* (James 1:22-24).

Forgetting what you look like would seem impossible. So too reading God's Word and not doing it. Being a "doer" of God's word simply means we get to "walk the talk!"

So how do you do that? I mean in a very real and practical way within the context of your everyday life?

Years ago a book was published that introduced a phrase to remind us to live like Jesus. It was simply, *"What would Jesus do?"* And not long after, to make certain we wouldn't forget, that phrase was popularized, abbreviated and initialed as W.W.J.D. on brightly colored rubber band bracelets.

Of course, wearing one meant you automatically raised the level of expectations around you. It was like wearing a billboard shouting out, "Watch my every move cuz I live like Jesus!"

It's interesting to note that when you ask an unbeliever what they think of Jesus, they will describe in detail His selfless behavior and humble lifestyle. And they want to use Him as a comparison to you and your behavior and lifestyle to see if you look anything like Jesus.

Don't you just love that? Or does that realization frighten you?

How are you doing in looking like Jesus? Apart from wearing the bracelet, could someone who knows you well, look at your life and make the statement that you act like Jesus?

You would think that the more time you spent with Him, doing what He says, the more you would actually resemble Him. It would be said of you like it was said of the apostles as recorded in Acts, when they stood on trial before the Pharisees, *"They took note that they had been with Jesus"* (Acts 4:13).

I met someone years ago who desperately wanted to live the way he believed Jesus commanded His followers to live. He knew about Jesus and wanted to model his life after Him.

So he determined to live out everything he studied in Jesus' sermon on the mount as it's recorded in Matthew 5, 6 and 7. He even set as a goal that within one year's time he would master this life and look like Jesus.

Sounds ambitious and a bit noble doesn't it? I admired him for his tenacity, but felt bad for him when he quit on the whole thing, stating, "It's just not possible!"

And how true that is, especially if you try to live that way on your own, which, unfortunately, was the case with him. You see he did not really *know* Jesus. He had not yet surrendered his life so that the power of God could live through him.

Doing it in your own strength is like trying to endlessly tread water without a life preserver. You'll last for only so long and then give out from exhaustion.

No, *trying* to live like Jesus is simply not going to work. You don't have the internal strength to do it. Someone said, *"The Christian life is not an **imitation** of the life of Christ. It is a **participation** in His life."*

Bam! There it is. Want to live like Jesus? Let go. Continually surrender your own ways and let His Spirit live His life in and through you.

If you do, then you will gladly embrace the command of Jesus. And he makes it real simple by summarizing it in Matthew 22:37-39 ... *"Love God with everything in you and love others as yourself."*

And in your everyday exchanges with the people around you, simply do what my dad said would make life a lot easier ... "Keep the Golden Rule!"

Or as Jesus put it ... *"Do to others whatever you would like them to do to you. This is the essence of all that is taught in the Law and the prophets"* (Matthew 7:12).

So you already know how that one plays out because all of us know exactly how we want to be treated by others.

Now go and do the same.

5

Don't Go It Alone.

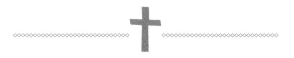

I'm a guy who, probably like you, prefers action movies. My favorites almost always seem to be battles of war based on true stories, such as *Private Ryan, Band of Brothers, Blackhawk Down* and *300* to name a few.

While I'm sure that I vicariously put myself in the movie as one of the diehard heroes willing to give my life for someone else, the bigger theme is that it takes a team to get it done.

You may have seen the acronym T-E-A-M, which stands for Together Everyone Achieves More. Kind of corny, but very true. None of the missions in each of these stories would have been accomplished if it were just one man attempting to do it all by himself.

I can guarantee, as good as the Chicago Bulls' Michael Jordan was in his prime back in the day, he still needed four other teammates on the court to win a game.

So it is with you, I mean *us*, that is!

You simply should not and cannot go through the battles of life without the support of other men. Guys who will have your back.

But the reality is, very few men are in that kind of *band of brothers* relationship with a group of men whom they can trust.

So, two questions for you:
1. Why is that?
2. Who's got your back?

As I mentioned at the outset, men are confused as to who they are, who they're "supposed" to be, and how that plays out in everyday life. Unfortunately, without some role models, men are left trying to figure it all out on their own.

So where do we go to see how a band of brothers live it out? And how do you make certain you are in relationship with a true band of brothers, someone who's got your back?

First let me clarify something. There are at least two categories of men who can form a band of brothers.

There are those who are *of the world*, concerned only about how to satisfy their own needs and advance their own cause. And there are those who are *spiritual* and *Kingdom-minded*, intent on advancing God's cause here on earth.

The worldly ones get together primarily for selfish purposes, to have some fun and get their own needs met. I have a friend who leans heavily on his buddies for companionship. But while he longs to have a deeper, more meaningful relationship, he ends up staying on the surface. They watch sports, play video games, drink and basically share stories about women they use or wish they could use.

This is a *pseudo* band of brothers because there is no higher cause they are living for, and in truth, are mostly buddies for the sake of just hanging out. They feel safe because they share common interests, but can't convert those interests into meaningful contributions for good. And when push comes to shove, they usually put themselves first and not their buddy.

The other category of men are a *true* band of brothers because they are spiritually-minded and intent on living out their faith as a true follower of Jesus. They are mission-minded, helping each other practice what they believe. And they are always on the lookout for others who need that same kind of help.

These are the men who, when they get together, study the Bible to see what God has to say about how to live their lives. They pray together. They talk through their struggles, their questions, their fears, and they celebrate their victories. And yes, they have fun and genuinely enjoy one another's company.

There is an authentic, unbreakable commitment to each other that assures each one that they are in this faith walk together and have each other's back.

Within days of my conversion to Christ, I was blessed to attend a church where men discipled new believers like me. From that point on, I knew I needed and could count on a band of brothers who had my back. In one of our groups, there is a core of eight men who have met together every week for over 25 years to study the Bible, pray together and walk through all of life's experiences.

So where are you today in relation to a band of brothers? Do you have brothers whom you know for certain have your back?

If you do, congratulations, don't stop!

If you don't, make it your top priority. Because if you don't have a band of brothers to walk it out with, you will fail. You cannot grow and you will not be effective in your faith without help from other men. Don't let yourself be fooled into thinking you are strong enough and dedicated enough on your own.

The 12 disciples of Jesus needed each other. Even Jesus himself was not a maverick, but lived it out with his band of brothers. **Men who love Jesus and want to follow Him simply need other men who love Jesus.**

If I sound like I'm harping on this, it's because I am. I've seen too many men wash out on the slippery slopes that challenge their faith. They start out strong but hold onto their independence, believing it is a sign of strength. Too afraid to show weakness, they end up becoming weaker by trying to go it alone.

In contrast, I have seen and experienced for myself the strength that comes when godly men are in relationship with other godly men. They get stronger as they walk it out together, encouraging and challenging each other.

So, what is stopping you? Hopefully it's not your pride. If, on the other hand, you're just not sure how to plug in with other godly men, then let me give you a couple of suggestions.

❐ First and foremost, make certain you are plugged into a Bible-believing, gospel-preaching church. If your church does not have a program for discipling men, then you have two choices:

1. Leave that church and find one that does.
2. Start a men's group yourself with the blessing of the pastor and elders.

It can be as simple as picking a night of the week or an early morning and inviting men to gather to study the Bible and help each other walk out their faith.

❐ Or you can do what I did over two decades ago, and that is to simply invite a handful of friends with whom you want to study the Bible. This does not mean each one of them must be mature in their faith and deeply rooted in the Scriptures. However, you do need a core of at least two to three guys along with yourself who are grounded in their faith and can help teach and disciple the others.

Regardless of whether you find a men's group in your church or start your own, there are plenty of resources to draw upon. While our men's group have used a variety of resources over the years, our mainstay is simply the Bible. We take a book of the Bible and walk through a portion each week to find out what is on God's heart and how we can apply His principles as followers of Jesus.

❐ Another great way to bond with a band of brothers is to go to a men's retreat or even a missions trip. This past year, I had the awesome privilege of joining a small group of men from our church's "Extreme Team." We backpacked into remote villages in the Himalayas to bring the gospel to the unreached.

It was one of the toughest challenges I've faced, physically, mentally and spiritually. But sharing the gospel of Jesus with people who have never heard of him, made me realize how God can use us if we are willing. This was a one of a kind experience and it bonded us together as men who will follow Jesus anywhere!

There are no shortages of ideas and opportunities for you to take advantage of if you are committed to go on your spiritual journey with other like-minded men.

Here are just a few of many great resources for men who are looking to join other men in becoming more like Jesus.

» Every Man a Warrior –

www.everymanawarrior.com

This is a ministry started by Lonnie Berger for the purpose of helping men succeed in life through a foundation in faith. The foundation of their ministry is a three-book study based on biblical principles that cover everything a man needs to know about walking with God, marriage and raising children, money, sex, work, hard times and how to make your life count. There are a total of 27 lessons filled with insights and practical applications.

» Bible Study Fellowship -

www.bsfinternational.org

This is the world's largest Bible study that meets weekly in small groups of 10-12 men who want to learn from God's Word. The studies are opportunities for you to question, discuss, listen, learn, and then apply the truths from the Bible.

» Ransomed Heart -

www.ransomedheart.com

This is undoubtedly one of the most comprehensive and impactful men's ministries you could possibly hope for. It was started by John Eldredge with his classic book Wild at Heart. If you've never read it and gone through the accompanying field manual, you are missing out. It will give you insights on what it means to be a man in relationship with God, men and women. You can also find on their website everything from podcasts, books and videos, to information on men's retreats and small groups.

» Marked Men for Christ -

www.markedmenforchrist.org

This is a new kind of men's ministry using powerful strategies that are proving to build stronger men for Christ from the inside out.

With such great resources available at our fingertips, along with so many others not mentioned here, there simply is no excuse for not recruiting and implementing help. My hope and prayer for you is that you don't delay for one day longer, but you commit to finding or forming a band of brothers and make it a priority in your life.

☐ Take a moment right now, or schedule time on your calendar, to outline the action steps you will take to get plugged in.

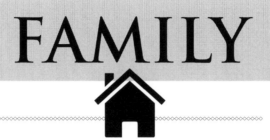

FAMILY

MERRIAM-WEBSTER DICTIONARY DEFINITION:

1 a: the basic unit in society traditionally consisting of two parents rearing their children
also: any of various social units differing from but regarded as equivalent to the traditional family

"As the family goes, so goes the nation and so goes the whole world in which we live."
- John Paul II

1

Identify Your Family Relationships

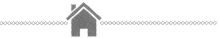

Years ago it was pretty easy to define family. It simply meant a dad and mom and their kids. In today's world, family has a much broader definition. It's all about *inclusion*.

I won't get into all of the complexities of the politically correct new definitions for family. For our purposes, we're just going to consider family in a more traditional manner.

This could include you being a son, a father, a husband, a grandfather. Or depending on your stage in life, a combination of all those.

The main focus in this section will be primarily for men who are sons, husbands and fathers. However, if you are single, please keep reading because there will be applications for you as you prepare for marriage and being a father.

Family was God's idea.

Think about it for a minute. When God created man (Adam) He decided it was not good for the man to be alone. So He created a woman (Eve, a helpmate) suitable to come alongside Adam in life. (See Genesis 2:18.)

God made each of them in His own image. Not physically and biologically, but having the same internal makeup such as a spirit, a mind, free will and the desire to love and be loved.

But God is not a man. And God is not a woman. God is an unembodied Spirit, both equally man and woman, living within a supernatural perfected state.

So if He wanted to, He could have created us in the same way, sharing both genders equally within the same human frame. But He didn't. He created male and female, two vastly different genders who are not only different in their physiological make-up, but quite opposite in the way they think and act.

And perhaps the more obvious reason for the differences between the sexes is for the purpose of procreation. God created the beautiful gift of sex between a man and a woman not only for sharing intimacy, but also for making babies.

How else can we perpetuate the human race?

Therefore we have families with a mom, a dad and children. Of course for you as a man, that means you are by default a son, possibly a brother, perhaps a husband and father and maybe even a grandfather. The reality is, you had no choice but to be part of a family, regardless of whether it was or is the ideal.

I have a brother-in-law who grew up in a large family that was a positive, nurturing, adventurous family with lots of uncles and aunts and married couples that stayed together. Many in their family were gifted with the intelligence and education to pursue careers in medicine. They modeled what it means to be Christ-followers and were known by their love, patience, kindness and commitment to family.

But let's be honest, that's more the exception than the rule. Most of us experienced varying degrees of dysfunction in the family we grew up in. And if you are married and have children, it is quite possible that some of what you experienced is being repeated.

I realize that your perception is subject to your interpretation of dysfunction and can be easily distorted based on unresolved issues. You may see yourself as a victim and indeed may have been or are being victimized by the sins of family members. You may be stuck in holding onto hurts that have caused fear, resentments and the justification to ignore, reject (disown) or retaliate.

So it would seem to make sense to run from instead of toward a family where there is hurt, bad role modeling and disillusionment.

But you have to make a choice in how you think about it.

Either God made a horrible mistake, or by design you were placed in that family for a reason and God can deepen your relationship with Him in spite of the dysfunction. He can bring good from anything and make the experience purpose-filled.

So take a moment and think about your family and your place in that family as a man, whether a son, husband and/or father. And if you are single, and marriage seems a long way off or maybe not at all for you, you are still a son, which means you have family.

☐ On the next page, write down your experience in family, the one you grew up in and the one you're currently part of. Identify whatever it is that needs your attention as you acknowledge and resolve the following:

- The good

- The bad

- The redeemable

One of the more challenging areas of life, is to know how to live purposely, joyfully and effectively within your family. That can be done more easily when we understand and own our role within the family.

2

Own Your Role as a Son

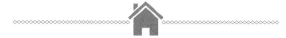

This is the common denominator for each of us because you have or had a father and a mother. If your parent(s) are still living, the good news is there's still time to carry out your role as a good son, showing love and honor to your parents.

Now it probably goes without saying that few sons would make claim to have grown up in the perfect family. Oh sure, there are a few exceptions, like the Beaver Cleaver TV family where June (the stay-at-home mom) always wore a dress, kept the house immaculate and baked cookies. And Ward (the professional, hard working, breadwinner dad) was almost always right and gave perfect advice to his sons and wife.

But that probably wasn't your family. In fact, maybe yours was the complete opposite and off the charts in chaos, dysfunction and pain. Nevertheless, as a son, you had to relate to a mom and a dad and you learned whatever it was they modeled for you.

The old adage, "More is caught than taught," is certainly true in a family. And to this day, be it good stuff or not so good stuff, you're default button is set to act out what you saw lived out in your home.

You may have had one parent absent from the home, or a chemically dependent parent, or a workaholic parent, or an abusive one, or a narcissistic, self-centered and unloving parent who modeled all the wrong things.

There are a host of behaviors that may have hurt you or negatively influenced you.

But here's the catch. Regardless of how things went growing up, as an adult son, you are still to honor your father and mother. That's not my idea, but God's, as He stated in the fifth commandment; *"Honor your father and your mother, then you will live a long and full life in the land the LORD your God is giving you"* (Exodus 20:12).

Notice that God gave no exceptions. He didn't say that if one or both of them were really bad parents, then you can just go ahead and ignore this commandment. Honoring a "bad" parent doesn't mean you approve or embrace their bad behavior. It doesn't mean you enable them or put yourself in a position of allowing continued mistreatment of you as their son.

You can still honor them by giving recognition and respect to their *position* as a mother or a father. And take note of something very important regarding God's commandment. This is the only commandment accompanied with a promise. Read it again.

"Honor your father and your mother, then you will live a long and full life in the land the LORD your God is giving you" (Exodus 20:12)

Do you want to live a good long life? Honor your parents. It's not only your responsibility, but can be a privilege with a great outcome attached to it.

I'm convinced that one of the reasons my dad lived to the age of 91 and my mom, currently 92, lived long lives, is because of the way they showed honor to their parents. And they showed honor via practical acts of love.

For example, after my mom's dad passed away, my dad took on the role of provider and protector for grandma. He helped her with every area of life. Whether he had the time for it or whether he felt like it, he honored her. My mom also checked in with grandma twice a day, and spent a lot of time with her, helping her with everything from the wash to grocery shopping.

It's just what families did for each other. And their example of how to honor parents showed me and my siblings the way it was done.

So in the two years before my own dad passed, we adult children had tremendous opportunities to love and help him in practical ways. And today we continue honoring my mom by caring for her every need. It is truly an honor and a privilege and I am expecting (while not deserving, mind you) a long life in return!

Now, a few practical suggestions of how you as a son, can show honor to your parents.

❐ Forgive, set them free, and be free.
We have all sinned, including your parents. Those sins, shortcomings and mistakes may have caused you pain to varying degrees. Forgive them, even as you yourself have been forgiven. That is the law of Christ.

❐ Reconcile.
If there is a need for reconciliation, to the degree that it's possible for you, reach out and reconcile. God will honor your efforts and you can trust Him for the outcome.

❐ Communicate often.

Nothing brings greater assurance to a parent that you love them, than a personal visit. Spend time with them. Do it as often as possible. Certainly, phone calls on a frequent basis are the next best thing in expressing love. (I know this probably goes without saying, but love is only authenticated in actions, not feelings.)

❐ Create ways to serve them.

Not sure what they need? Ask. As your parents grow older, they become less able to do the things that were once easy. I can promise that if you have not yet experienced the phenomena of role reversal with your parents, you will. Just like when you were a child and needed help with the simple things of life, as your parents age, they revert back to childlikeness and you become the parent and caregiver. Do it with joy, patience and respect, and count it a privilege to show honor in that way.

3

Own Your Role as a Husband (or Husband-to-Be)

First and foremost, I'm going with the assumption that you are committed to making your marriage revolve around your relationship with Christ. If you don't, the chances are slim that your marriage will last, or at the least, be what God intended for you.

The Bible calls it being "equally yoked." When oxen were strapped together to pull the plow, they were harnessed to a wooden yoke. You can imagine how difficult it would be to have one large ox and one small one yoked together. That's not going to work too well, and it certainly won't end up plowing a straight line.

You must not compromise when it comes to being spiritually yoked. Putting the Lord first in your marriage and walking out the Christian life together, all but guarantees you will grow together and can get through anything that is thrown in your way.

Here is a caution for "husbands-to-be."

You must not compromise in the area of pre-marital sex either. Put simply: do NOT have sexual intimacy before you are married. Why not? Because in the Bible God says it is a sin.

And why is it a sin? Because it keeps you from Him and hurts your soul. Premarital sex does not require any commitment. It costs you nothing and gains you temporary pleasure while forfeiting your soul.

Sexual intimacy is a gift, created by God so that the two of you can become "one flesh."

It is to be honored and valued and held in reserve until you are willing to commit yourself to her in a marriage for life.

The role of being a husband is by far one of the greatest challenges for men today.

Because in our self-absorbed, what's-in-it-for-me society, being a "godly" husband requires death! Death to your self-centeredness and selfish demands to be first.

Again, that's not my idea but God's, written in His Word as instructions for us. *"Husbands love your wives just as Christ loved the church and gave up his life for her…"* (Ephesians 5:25).

Indeed, Jesus Christ laid down His life for you. Are you willing to do the same for your wife?

If not, make it right. Don't put it off. If you truly put her first, ahead of you, in everything, you will not only meet your wife's needs, you will capture her heart. And a wife's captured heart means you will be more loved and respected than you can imagine.

But there are three realities that will challenge you.

1. Putting her first requires the genuine want to, not the have to.

Jesus did not *have* to die for you. He *wanted* to because He knew the outcome would be intimacy between you and God. While it may take intentional effort on your part, trying to force yourself into it will not work, and you will fail because she knew you were forcing it. And you will feel misunderstood, unappreciated and sorry for yourself.

You can literally create the new motive of want to over have to by focusing on the outcome. You want to have her love and respect you and this is the way to get it. God knows what is best for you (and her) and it's why He gave you this instruction and example through Jesus. He will make good on it for you as you trust Him and follow through on it.

2. It will take time to build up a proven track record.

We are accustomed to getting what we want, when we want it, in our on-demand world. Anything that takes time and requires patience is a very foreign thing to us. But living this out consistently is key. As your wife begins to experience being put first, you will by default raise the bar on her expectations.

However, you will likely stumble and resort back to selfishness, which she will immediately notice. You will be tempted to give up on it. Don't do it! Stay in there. Fight for it. Fight for her. Pick yourself back up and prove to yourself that you really can die to your selfish wants. It takes time. It takes practice and perseverance. And it will absolutely take something greater than yourself to pull it off.

3. You are completely powerless to do this on your own.

I don't think you have to be convinced of how seemingly impossible it is to live unselfishly, always putting your wife first. To have any degree of success requires a source of power way beyond your own capabilities. It doesn't matter if you have the discipline and perseverance of a Navy SEAL.

In your own strength you will fail.

It takes supernatural power. And that is why, when you fully and consistently surrender your life to the Lord, He, and not you, will be in charge. It's not you sharing the throne with Jesus, but Jesus, through His Holy Spirit, running the show.

Jesus said, *"Apart from me you can do nothing" (John 15:5). But in Christ, "you can do all things"* (Philippians 4:13). If you believe that and act on it, you will have the power you need to live unselfishly and become more and more like Christ.

Of course you agree, but lest all this gets stuck in your head, you have to become practical in the everyday outworking of being an unselfish husband.

First things first.

Check yourself out on each one of the following items. Next to each one, write down a score between 1 and 10 on how you're doing. A score of 1 means you're not doing it at all, and 10 means your wife is going to write a book about you and how she married the perfect husband! Anything under a 5 means you need to give it *immediate* attention.

After you complete this exercise, for each item write down at least one thing you can do today to bump up that score.

❏ **Acknowledge that your chief role as husband is to protect and provide.**
This is what men do. The first line of defense in protecting and providing for your wife, is to lead her spiritually. That means you initiate prayer together, reading the Bible, going to church, serving the Lord and modeling the spirit-filled life of being a Christ-follower. If you're not sure about that responsibility, take time to talk to godly men around you whom you believe are living this out, to help you understand and commit to that role.

☐ Learn her love language.

Stop trying to love your wife the way you're comfortable loving her. Love her the way she needs to be loved. I had a wise and seasoned husband tell me that his marriage completely turned around after he discovered this simple truth. "God wants to love my wife His way but through me." So on occasion, I ask the Lord how He wants me to show HIS love to her today.

☐ Embrace your differences.

As John Eldridge teaches, "She is not a puzzle to solve but a mystery to explore." Stop trying to make her like you. What a disaster that would be. God's Word said He made your wife as a "suitable helper." In the original language, a helper is one who fills up the gaps. Yep, you got gaps and your beautiful and very different-than-you wife can help fill those in, if you will let her. Which, by the way, will inevitably make her a lot more content as she is given opportunity to live out what she is naturally designed to be and do.

☐ Let her be right.

Even when you're pretty certain she is wrong, don't let on. Unless it is some life-changing topic, what's the big deal? It's only your pride that gets bruised when you have to be right. Instead, yield the floor and give it to her.

My friend, Stewart, had been married for over 20 years. It was an "okay" marriage but fraught with arguments. They were the classic "Bickersons." Each one of them more stubborn than the other and unrelenting in needing to be right. Finally, Stewart decided that with God's help, he would lay down his life (rights) and let his wife be right – all the time.

At first it was excruciating because he felt that as a man he should never cave in. Then he realized that the meekness of Jesus was a greater strength on the inside of him than anything on the outside. It wasn't long and he not only got free from having to be right, he felt joy whenever he could sincerely tell his wife, "You know, I think you're right, honey."

The result? The arguments stopped and her love and respect for him went through the roof. And it wasn't long after, that she gladly deferred to him, even when initially she thought he was wrong.

☐ Don't let the sun go down on your anger.

The apostle Paul gave us those instructions in Ephesians 4:26 as a way of helping us prevent deterioration in our marriage. If a grievance by you or your spouse is not resolved by the time you fall asleep, it gets locked in and can sour into bitterness and resentment. Those are two sins that can have permanent consequences.

While my mom and dad didn't have a marriage free of problems, dad was the one who made certain they didn't go to bed angry. Regardless of how you feel, keep short accounts and go to bed free of anger. It will reinforce your love commitment and allows you to start the next day with a fresh perspective.

☐ Do what comes *unnatural* for you.

When certain requests come up from your wife, sometimes they are the exact opposite of what you want. You know what I'm referring to. Things like shopping together in the mall, watching chick flicks, listening to ALL the details as she gives an account of her day, letting her pick the vacation spot, giving her preference in home make-over projects, and actually asking her for a Honey-do list and then doing it. It's not natural. It's not easy. But do it and there will be HUGE payoffs for you.

☐ Romance her like you did before you caught her.

Yep. Men are hunters and you know what it took to get the trophy. When you were in hot pursuit before you married, she knew that your universe revolved around her. You romanced her in creative ways that came natural for you. You never thought twice about putting her needs first, spending time with her or cherishing her. So you obviously have it in you.

Why then, does any husband stop doing that once the honeymoon is over?

Maybe we get too comfortable, take things for granted, or get bored and lazy. Fight against it. You MUST keep things fresh and alive in your marriage. Find ways to make love to your wife all day long, *without having sex*. And when your lovemaking does culminate in sexual intimacy, it will be the true definition of, *"and the two shall become one"* (Matthew 19:5).

☐ Don't go it alone.

Get help. There simply are no excuses for not knowing what to do as a husband, or how to do it. There are numerous resources for men who want to know how to commit to becoming a husband that exemplifies the true meaning of unconditional love. Start by looking for that man in your network that has a great marriage. Ask him to help you become a better husband and start modeling what he does. And remember, if you are in a small group with a band of brothers, it's guaranteed they will be eager to help you, pray with you and encourage you.

Here are a few resources that can help:

» **Ransomed Hearts** - www.ransomedheart.com
Start with John Eldredge's book, Wild at Heart, the standard for what makes up a man and how he can live out his full manness, including being the husband he was meant to be.

» **Love and Respect** - www.loveandrespect.com
Get a good foundation by reading the book, Love and Respect, by Dr. Emerson Eggrichs. This is a classic among marriage books, and shows a husband how to live out his role from a biblical position.

» **His Needs/Her Needs** - www.hisneedsherneeds.com
First read the book by Dr. Willard Harley, His Needs, Her Needs.

This will give you practical insights for understanding your mate's needs. Through their books and videos, Dr. Harley and his wife Joyce, provide eye-opening and convincing insights as to the real needs of each spouse, and how to go about meeting them.

» Marriage Encounter - www.marriage-encounter.org

These are weekend marriage conferences that give spouses an opportunity to grow in their marriage through open and honest communication, face-to-face sharing, and heart-to-heart encounters in a comfortable, relaxed setting. They have an incredible track record of strengthening and restoring marriages.

4

Own Your Responsibility to Love Unconditionally

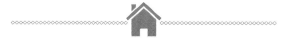

"Above all, love each other deeply, because love covers a multitude of sins." 1 Peter 4:8 (NIV)

To the degree that you carry out your role as husband, you better your chances of maintaining a happy and peaceful marriage with a wife who loves and respects you and meets your needs in return.

But what if you started out too late in the process and there is irreversible damage? What if no matter what you try at this point, it doesn't seem to be enough and she is finished with the marriage.

Or on the other hand, even after you have given it your very best effort, you have an unhappy, hurting wife who in turn hurts and rejects you.

Human nature means a sinful nature and a choice to yield to it or to the Spirit of Jesus. You can control that process within yourself, but not your wife.

She may have life-long, unresolved issues that she brought with her into your marriage. They may have impacted her to the point of causing such pain, confusion and even dysfunction, that no matter what you do, it can't fix the problem or heal her soul.

What do you do? How do you handle something you have no control over?

Surrender to Jesus. Stay faithful. Love her unconditionally. Live out your role as a husband blamelessly. Don't defend or justify or retaliate. Sound too simplistic? As a follower of Jesus, what are your other options?

If she leaves, you let her go. If she divorces you, you still love her unconditionally and you let God sort out the details. If, over time, reconciliation is no longer an option, you move on. If you had children together, you work tirelessly as a single dad, modeling unconditional love for their mother. You don't ever, ever bad-mouth her. You find the good in her and always point them to that.

Sound impossible? Indeed it is. In your own strength, that is. But you are a man of God, surrendered to His Spirit and filled with His love, so that it effortlessly flows through you and out to her and your children. You deny your own feelings and you do the right thing at all times and in all situations.

I know a man who married his childhood sweetheart at the age of 20. But he was immature, self-centered and ill-equipped to be a good husband. After six years and two children, his wife left him for another man. While going through the most excruciatingly painful experience of his life, God reached out and grabbed hold of him. His life was completely changed from the inside out as he surrendered his life to Jesus.

However, it was too late to save his marriage. But he made a decision that it was never too late to show unconditional love, especially to the wife of his youth, even though she was now married to her lover.

As a single dad with two little ones he made sure his daughters would see unconditional love and forgiveness in his words, thoughts and actions toward their mother.

He remained single for ten years and made a commitment that as a father and former husband, he would live out his faith walk with purity and integrity. The pain of that loss, and especially the way in which it happened, could have left him bitter and resentful. Instead, as a committed follower of Jesus, he depended on and trusted God's Spirit for the power needed to live in love, grace and freedom.

5

Own Your Role
as a Father

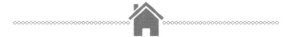

As a man, you were created with the wiring to be a father. It's woven into your manhood DNA.

You had a dad so you already have a taste of what that role entails. Regardless of whether your dad was a good dad or not, or absent altogether, as a man you have within you a built-in mechanism for fatherhood.

And because each of us are uniquely created by God, He has a claim on being our true, lasting and perfect Father.

Perhaps you've heard it said that your image of God as a father was shaped by your relationship with your earthly dad. That's probably very true.

If your dad was patient, compassionate, kind, present, and all of the other attributes and behaviors that make up a loving father, then your image of God as a father was well-shaped.

But if your dad was impatient, stern, mean, neglectful and a host of other negative traits, then your image of God as a father has been deeply flawed.

And if there was no dad in your life as you grew up, your image of God can make it feel like God is not interested or never there for you.

Take a moment right now and pause to reflect on your relationship with your dad. Better yet, write down the good, the bad and the "I just don't get it" stuff about your dad.

The good:

The bad:

The "I just don't get it" stuff:

Now, thank God for the good. Forgive your dad for the bad. And for the stuff he did that never made sense, surrender it to God and let Him sort it out.

Remember that we are biased in our assessment of our fathers. We typically judge them harshly because of their imperfections and our unrealistic expectations. That's not an excuse for your dad's failures, just an explanation. Like you, he has a sinful nature and like you, he needs forgiveness.

Here's the good news; you can have an accurate picture of God as your Father if you will simply read His Word. Keep it simple by going to the Gospels and reading the accounts of how Jesus related to His heavenly Father whom He called Abba (Daddy). His Father is your Father, and Jesus models for you what that relationship can be like. The more you draw from your relationship with God as your Father, the better you become as a dad.

Not a dad yet? Single and not planning on getting married and having kids? Married but never had kids? It doesn't matter.

It can still all apply to you. Why? Because, whether or not you have biological children of your own, I can guarantee God will bring into your life someone who needs fathering. It might even be more than one person. Remember, that's part of your wiring and what God has already equipped you to be and do.

And if your "son" or "daughter" has not shown up yet, go find one!

Seriously. In our society today, there is a huge vacuum that exists in the hearts of fatherless children who are longing for a man to step up and take the place of a dad.

Start with your immediate family. Are you an uncle who's brother or brother-in-law is no longer present in the home? Step in and be more than just an uncle. Offer those kids the best of what a father could give.

No nephews or nieces? Look around in your church, or neighborhood, or work, and you will find single moms raising kids without a father. Perhaps he's deceased or divorced and has abandoned the kids. Fatherless children are out there and they need what you have.

So what exactly do you have and how do you use what you have to be a good father?

1. Commit to believing you have what it takes.
You have the same fatherhood potential as your Heavenly Father. You were made in His image and if you have surrendered your life to Him and received His Holy Spirit into you, then you already have all that you need to be a good dad.

BELIEVE IT. OWN IT. BE IT. USE IT!

2. Speak good things into your children.
Believe the best about them and for them at every age. Their self-image is shaped by what they believe you think of them. Speak encouraging words of confidence and affirmation into your children until they believe you believe in them.

My brother, Brad, and his wife are classic examples of how well this works. They poured positive, confidence-building, verbal messages of non-stop affirmation into their three sons.

To be honest, some of us rolled our eyes over what we thought was a bit overboard. "Good job going to the toilet good son. Great job walking through the house instead of running. Excellent way to share your toys good, good son!"

I mean to tell you it absolutely hardwired into those boys a good self-image so that when discipline came, they still knew they were loved.

And today, all three of their adult sons have for many years been serving (with confidence) as high ranking Marines with impactful levels of responsibilities. That's the payoff for speaking good things into your children's lives.

❑ Write out three statements you can verbally repeat to each child that convinces them you believe the best in them.

1.

2.

3.

3. Remember, more is caught than taught.
They are watching you and they will imitate you. Your lifestyle, attitudes and behaviors are being etched into their hearts. You already know this from your own experience with your own dad. And more than likely, you have on numerous occasions caught yourself saying and doing the same things your dad did.

Be aware then, your kid is very likely going to turn out like you, so make it count. Repeat for your kids all the good your dad did for you. Delete any of the bad you experienced so you don't let it get passed down to your children. Like it or not, your dad modeled for you his version of how to be a dad. As an adult you know what worked and what didn't. Value it and learn from it.

❏ Make a list of what you want to imitate from your dad's parenting.

❏ Make another list of the things you don't want to imitate.

4. Teach them about God and His ways.

You are creating their image of God, so raise them with an awareness of who He is. God is the perfect Father and your children need to know Him and how He relates as a dad. The truth of who He is and how He acts is in His Word.

Read and discuss the Bible together. Show them what He reveals about Himself, His character and His actions. If you're pointing them in the right direction, they will see His Fatherly love in His compassion, mercy, forgiveness, provision, intervention, authority and power.

Of course, the more you do this, it's like holding up a mirror to see what you're reflecting, and will challenge you to become a godly dad. Take advantage of the teaching moments with your kids throughout the day. Use illustrations or life examples, and show them how to apply those examples to their lives.

When my daughters were quite young we loved to go out hiking. One day the path we were on split into a fork, with one path wider and an easier decline, and the other one much narrower and steep.

I paused at the top and told them how Jesus taught us that there are two paths we can follow in life. One is wide and easy, which everyone wants to take. But this path leads to trouble. The other one is narrow and very few want to take it, but Jesus says this is the one to stay on if we follow Him. We gave examples of what happens in our lives depending on the path we take. When I asked them which one we should go down, they both enthusiastically shouted, "This one dad!" I was proud to say we took the steep, narrow one. It was a great life lesson!

"Teach them (God's words) to your children, talking about them when you sit at home and when you walk along the road, when you lie down and when you get up." Deuteronomy 11:19 (NIV)

❏ Think of at least one lesson each of your children need to learn. Then write out a few ideas on how you want to illustrate it and use God's Word as your authority.

5. Discipline your children.
But make sure you understand its meaning and purpose. You've heard it said, "Spare the rod, spoil the child." That's true, but so misunderstood.

According to the Oxford Dictionary, discipline means "to train one to obey rules or a code of behavior and using correction or punishment for disobedience"

But far too often a dad who forgets the training part of discipline can quickly react in anger and lash out with instant punishment. That's the easy way out and not good. It takes work and it takes time to train, but the end result is much better with a more permanent outcome. *"Train up a child in the way he should go and when he is older he will not depart from it."* Proverbs 22:6 (ESV)

❏ How are you currently disciplining your children?

❏ How can you make it an effective training instead of simply reaction and punishment?

6. Spend one-on-one time with each child.

There simply is no excuse not to do this. Forget about the work/job/career excuse-making. Your time with your kids will fly by and all your good intentions of doing things with them will come to nothing.

You MUST intentionally, willfully, uncompromisingly *make*, not *take*, time for your children.

Go out with them. Talk, listen, share from your own life, involve them in things like work, sports, hobbies. Let them shadow you for a day. You don't always have to be the big entertainer. Just spend time with them.

My son-in-law has eight children! Yes, my daughter's husband. So I am a blessed grandfather! He deliberately plans time with each of them so he can give all of himself. He has huge responsibilities at work and at home. Nevertheless, he knows the importance of investing in his kids and reassuring each one that they are equally important to him. So he finds simple ways to involve them in every aspect of his life.

❏ Stop what you're doing for a moment and put on your schedule a time you will do something one-on-one with each of your children. Do it right now before you go any further.

7. Don't just *know* it, *show* it.

Put on display, often and in front of your children, affection, respect, unconditional love and fierce loyalty to their mother. Model for them how a man treats a woman and how a husband treats a wife. Never treat her harshly. Avoid being impatient with her. Let them watch and listen as you converse with her. Don't argue in front of the children. Compliment her in front of them. Model manly gestures toward her. Yes, go around to her side of the car and open the door for her. Carry all the groceries in. Simple things. Let them see you smile at her, even flirt. Explain why you still take her on dates and like to be alone with her.

Help them understand why she takes first place in your life.

❏ Commit to at least three things you will do, starting today, to show your children how a man treats a woman.

8. Bless them every day.

There is tremendous power in blessings. The Bible gives numerous examples of God extending His words of blessings, as well as others speaking out blessings, especially over their children.

> Spoken blessings build confidence, encouragement and faith in those being blessed. A blessing leaves the one being blessed with a sense of expectation that what was spoken over them will actually happen.

Try it out. You can literally put your hand on the head of each child, either in the morning or evening before bed, and pray out loud a blessing over them.

❏ Search the Bible for numerous examples of blessings. Here are just a few: (ESV)

- *"For you bless the righteous, O Lord; you cover him with favor as with a shield"* (Psalm 5:12).

- *"Let the favor of the Lord our God be upon us, and establish the work of our hands..."* (Psalm 90:17).

- *"For I know the plans I have for you declares the Lord, plans for welfare and not for evil, to give you a future and a hope"* (Jeremiah 29:11).

- *"And God is able to bless you abundantly, so that in all things at all times having all that you need, you will abound in every good work"* (2 Corinthians 9:8).

- *"Surely your goodness and love will follow me all the days of my life, and I will dwell in the house of the LORD forever"* (Psalm 23:6).

- *"The Lord bless you and keep you; the Lord make his face shine on you and be gracious to you; the Lord turn his face toward you and give you peace"* (Numbers 6:24-26).

❏ Check out this nine-minute video on YouTube.
Search for: Richard Brunton - *The Father's Blessing*.

❏ Write out your blessing and commit to repeating it out loud over your children every day.

9. You're never going to get it all right, so get help.
Don't be stubborn and prideful. You can do that when it comes to getting directions while driving, but not raising kids. There are kazillions of resources to teach you how to be a good dad with godly principles for raising your kids.

Here are a few to get you started:

» Focus on the Family -
www.focusonthefamily.com/parenting
Started by Dr. James Dobson, this is by far one of the best, time-tested and comprehensive ministries that will give you the insights and practical tools needed to help you raise godly children.

» Visionary Families -
www.visionaryfam.com
   Born out of the experience with his own family, Dr. Rob Rienow developed this ministry to help build strong families and equip parents to pass along faith and character to their children and grandchildren.

» 14 GOSPEL PRINCIPLES
That Can Radically Change Your Family -
www.paultripp.com/parenting
   Paul Tripp outlines 14 foundational principles centered on the gospel to help parents embrace a grand perspective of parenting overflowing with vision, purpose, and joy.

MY STORY AS A DAD.

I was a single dad for ten years, co-raising half-time my six-year-old daughter, Stephanie, and her three-month-old little sister, Angela. It was the highest privilege and calling of my life! They were my top priority.

I was absolutely certain that God entrusted them to me so that I could raise them up in the ways of the Lord and help expand his Kingdom with these two little disciples.

Every day on my knees I would thank God for them, surrender them back to Him, and promise that I would do everything humanly possible, but trust Him to do the impossible.

I made my share of mistakes, but always kept learning, growing and never stopped trying to be a better dad.

Today, my two adult daughters are my heroes and I continue to give them constant praise for who they are and how they live their lives.

They love God and as committed followers of Jesus, they are determined to raise up their children in the ways of the Lord. My greatest joy is seeing my 12 grandchildren learning what was passed down to their mothers. Only they are, of course, much better at it than I was. They are much more informed and have more practice with so many kids.

Besides managing their homes and working as entrepreneurs on a variety of ventures, they also homeschool their children. It's an all-out commitment, because they understand the privilege and responsibility God has given them as parents to make disciples, starting with their children.

And because more is caught than taught, this will have a ripple effect as their children are seeing it modeled, so they can in turn do the same when they become parents.

As a man and your brother on this faith journey with you, I am begging you to take your role as a father as the highest calling and privilege God has entrusted to you.

Take it seriously. Make it a matter of life and death for eternity.

Loving your children as God loves you and making disciples of Jesus is your legacy!

❒ What is your story as a dad and what legacy do you want to leave your children?

FITNESS

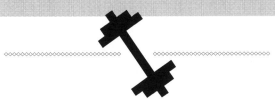

OXFORD LIVING DICTIONARIES DEFINITION:

1. the condition of being physically fit and healthy.
2. the quality of being suitable to fulfill a particular role or task.

FITNESS

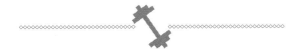

Did you catch definition #2?

Think about it for a moment. How many times do you feel like you are not suitable or equipped to fulfill a particular role or task?

What if we could change that by getting fit and staying that way?

The reality is, getting fit can be uncomfortable and most of us have become soft. We can't help it because we live in a time and place where the creature comforts we depend on have caused us to become resistant to being uncomfortable. In fact, why should we be uncomfortable when the goal is for the comforts surrounding us to make our lives easier and more efficient?

I rediscovered that reality when I went on a backpacking missions trek in the Himalayan mountains. We travelled for 40 hours to get there in cramped airline seats, and bounced around in a van for six hours on mountain trails. I slept on the ground with no air conditioning, no cell phones, no computers, no toilets, no showers and no clean clothes, and ate unfamiliar food. I was often hungry, tired and exhausted mentally, spiritually and physically, and was very uncomfortable.

If it weren't for the mental and spiritual prep, along with four months of physical training, I would not have had *the quality of being suitable to fulfill a particular role or task.*

You get the idea. There are so many challenges you face every day, that if you don't get in shape and toughen up, you will not be fit enough to carry out your roles or tasks. Learning how to be uncomfortable and pushing through the pain is a huge advantage in being and staying fit enough to handle anything that comes your way.

And of course, when we talk about fitness, it can and should include being fit in spirit, mind and body. In Section 1 we covered spiritual fitness, and will touch on being mentally fit later in this section.

But when it comes to physical fitness, it typically includes these components:

• Cardiorespiratory fitness
• Muscular strength
• Muscular endurance
• Body composition
• Flexibility and balance

So, as you look at that list, are you fit? Do you like the way you look? The way you feel? Are you in exactly the place you hoped to be with your health, wellness and physical shape? Do you implement a consistent, well-balanced, wholistic plan that gives you the energy, health and longevity that causes your doctor to scratch his head in amazement and ask you what you're doing to stay in such remarkable shape?

If yes, skip this next section cuz I got nothing new for you.

If no, you are NOT in the physical health and wellness place you want to be, ask yourself why not? It's probably a simple answer along the lines of:

• "I just don't have time."
• "I've tried everything and nothing works."
• "It's genetics and I have an unusually slow metabolism."
• "I don't know enough about it and don't know where to start."
• "It's just too hard and I'm fine the way I am."
• "I simply am not going to give up what I like to eat and I'm sure not going to sweat my butt off to lose a couple pounds!"

So, as you scan that list or add in other reasons why you're not in shape, you've basically chosen to believe lies, right? Is that too harsh? Okay then, consider them instead as excuses. Either way, those reasons are blocking your way and you can, and need to, knock down those barriers!

The first place to start is to get clear on exactly what you want for your health and fitness and *why* you want it.

That may sound too elementary, but if you don't have that clarity solidly locked in your head, then nothing I lay out for you will work and you will fail.

Getting and staying in shape starts with your mindset, in other words, what you believe and the commitment you will make to achieve it.

It requires you to be brutally honest with yourself and to own up to the consequences of not being healthy and fit.
The Bible says your body is a temple of the Holy Spirit. The Lord doesn't need you posing on the cover of Muscle and Fitness magazine, but He does expect you to treat your body with respect and to care for it.

"Don't you realize that your body is the temple of the Holy Spirit, who lives in you and was given to you by God? You do not belong to yourself..." (1 Corinthians 6:19).

"... I plead with you to give your bodies to God because of all he has done for you. Let them be a living and holy sacrifice—the kind he will find acceptable. This is truly the way to worship him" (Romans 12:1).

He has a purpose, plans and "good works" that He created you to carry out on His behalf. If you needlessly get sick, run out of energy, carry around extra weight that puts your health at risk, you potentially short circuit what God wants to do through you.

You know the feeling you get when you drive by a worn down, trashy looking, neighborhood that was not cared for? You know it doesn't have to be that way if they would just show a little respect and take care of their place.

Yet you can make excuses for neglecting your own body and complain about being overweight and out of shape. You already know what it costs you because you don't have the energy, strength or stamina to endure all that life throws at you.

The stresses of today takes a toll on you, and the longer you let your health go, the worse it gets as you age. At some point some men, maybe you, just give up and embrace their unhealthy, unfit condition.

That is so sad and so wrong.

It is never too late to get back in shape! Want to get inspired? Just do a quick search on the internet for elderly people who started working out and eating right later in life. Today, they are competing in races, bodybuilding, mountain climbing – you name it and they're doing it!

So can you! But you need to start out with enough reason and motivation to want to make the changes.

1

Determine *What* You Want and *Why*

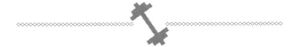

In fact, if you don't take a few minutes to write out your what and why, then you're still not fully committed to wanting change in your health and physical shape.

When you write down what you want, you lock it in and take the first step in making a commitment.

But don't be generic when writing it out.

In other words, "I want to look and feel better," doesn't really mean a lot without specific details of what that looks like for you.

So be as specific as you can when you think about what it is you actually want to look like and feel like for your health and fitness. For example, it could go along these lines.

I want to *look* better by:

• losing 20 lbs of fat, 3" off my waist.
• adding five lbs of muscle.
• having noticeably better muscular definition in my arms and legs and abs.

• having clear skin, clear eyes and a well-groomed appearance.
• standing and walking with an upright posture, shoulders back, head up, and displaying confidence in who I am.

I want to *feel* better by:

• consistently getting a deep, solid sleep of eight hours a night.
• eliminating the afternoon sleepy slump.
• functioning younger than my age by at least ten years.
• replacing the need for caffeine energy spikes and still have high sustainable energy.
• being able to feel a pump in my muscular structure.
• experiencing a peaceful anchoring in the middle of the daily stresses.

❐ **Write out how you want to look and what you want to feel like.**

❐ **Next pick a date when you're going to evaluate your results and get it on your calendar.**
This needs to be realistic. This is not the end-all of your health and wellness achievements. It is a journey. But there have to be milestones along the way that mark your progress or motivate you to go the next level. You may need to break things up in stages, but if you don't put markers to hit at specific dates, you will not make measurable progress.

So pick the dates and get them on your calendar!

☐ Now take a few minutes and write out your why.

Answering your *why* is truly the only way you have any hope of staying motivated to get in shape and stay healthy.

• *Why* do you want what you just wrote down about the way you want to look and feel?

• How will it make a difference for you today, in 90 days, and ten years from now?

• How will it make a difference for your family? For your work? For your self-image and ability to function at your maximum potential?

• How can pushing your body to do what is uncomfortable help you face other uncomfortable challenges in other areas of life?

• What difference will it make for you in realigning a healthy self-image?

• How will it energize and help motivate you to carry out the work God has given you to do?

Don't rush through this exercise. Whether you've done some of this before or never before, it's important at any age and stage in life to recalibrate so that you can continually improve your health and wellness.

God's Word says your body is a temple for His Holy Spirit to live within. Don't take this lightly. A temple is a sacred place dedicated for holiness, purity and worship. Your body is not to be worshipped, but to be indwelt by God Himself. You literally can be a vessel in which He can move around and accomplish His purposes through you.

If there is nothing restricting you, but you are *NOT* intentionally staying healthy, strong and in shape, you hamper your potential to function effectively.

Now hear me out on this. If you are in any way physically handicapped, it does not mean you are exempt from being a temple and a vessel for God to work through. A classic example is Helen Keller, who was deaf and blind, yet accomplished more in her 88 years than most fully functioning people could ever hope for.

There is a long list of heroes who have not viewed their disability as something to stop them from being productive and contributing to the betterment of others.

Joni Eareckson Tada, a quadriplegic since age 18, is a Christian author, speaker, artist, musician, radio host and international advocate for those with disabilities. She has inspired millions of people to love God and live out their potential.

Nick Vujicic, the man born with no arms and no legs is an evangelist, motivational speaker, author and founder of Life Without Limbs. He has shared his message of hope to millions, empowering them to overcome their challenges.

Sam Berns, the young man disabled with progeria who passed away at age 17, achieved his dreams and accomplished things in life that are still inspiring and motivating millions. Check out his TED talk: "My Philosophy for a Happy Life."

❏ **ACTION POINT**: To be inspired and motivated, take 30 minutes and check out their websites and videos. After viewing the way they live their lives, what's your excuse for not fully living out your potential?

❏ Write a one sentence statement about what you want to duplicate from each one of their examples.

2

Assess Your Current Condition

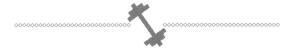

Assuming that you now have a stronger why, and know more specifically what you want for your health and fitness, it's time to determine your starting point.

This is simply an exercise for gathering data to assess your baseline wellness status. Knowing exactly where you are, compared to where you want to be, will help you set specific goals. This is absolutely crucial in helping you measure your progress and staying motivated to develop an ever-improving lifestyle.

❏ **ACTION POINT**: Take a notebook or use the space here to record the following data points. (Make several copies.) This will be your current status, or your BEFORE assessment.

Measure each body part every three weeks on a non-training day. Ensure that muscles are not flexed when you measure them, as this will produce an inconsistent result given there is usually a wide variation between individual, flexed body parts.

DATE	WEIGHT	BICEPS	FOREARMS	NECK	CHEST	WAIST	THIGHS	CALVES
		Left: Right:	Left: Right:				Left: Right:	Left: Right:
		Left: Right:	Left: Right:				Left: Right:	Left: Right:
		Left: Right:	Left: Right:				Left: Right:	Left: Right:
		Left: Right:	Left: Right:				Left: Right:	Left: Right:
		Left: Right:	Left: Right:				Left: Right:	Left: Right:
		Left: Right:	Left: Right:				Left: Right:	Left: Right:

On a scale of 1-10 rate your level of satisfaction for the following:

POSITIVE MENTAL ATTITUDE					
SPIRITUAL HEALTH					
OVERALL PHYSICAL HEALTH					
GROOMING HABITS					
PARTICIPATING IN SPORTS					
EATING HABITS					
SLEEP QUALITY					
CARDIO ABILITY					
DATE					

There may be other specific areas of your health, wellness and fitness that you want to assess. So I want to encourage you to take time now to write down everything you believe needs to be reevaluated. Obviously, it will be beneficial to write down those specific areas that need improvement. All of this will figure into your goal setting and planning as you take charge of maximizing your potential.

❒ **Critical areas of my health and wellness I need to reevaluate:**

3

Set Your Goals

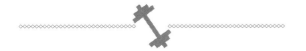

If you're accustomed to setting goals in your life, then you already know the value of writing down specific things you aim to achieve. And you also know that without a specific plan that includes a timeline, those goals are seldom achieved. If setting goals is new to you, then you are in for a great experience of developing what can become lifetime habits.

Some people refer to their goals as dreams, visions or hopes. However, in my opinion, that makes it all too vague. It's easy to lose motivation if there is something that always seems to lie just beyond your reach.

But with goals, it becomes a simple matter of specifying what it is you want to accomplish, and when it's going to be achieved. You put together a plan outlining the details of what it will take over time to measure the outcome.

Now, I know that some people buck up against setting goals as being too restrictive, not allowing them to flow in the Spirit and live in the moment. Some may feel that this is more of a 21st century, western cultural thing. Or that it has no biblical roots and therefore is not all that relevant.

Call them whatever you will, but everyone has goals. It might not be anything formal or anything you're consciously aware of, but you had a goal of waking up today, getting to work on time, staying on your side of the road, doing certain work tasks, feeding your body, going to bed and sleeping, etc.

Maybe you are not consciously setting or reaching those daily routine goals, but in practice you are already accustomed to doing them. Now you're being challenged to get much more intentional and specific about setting measurable goals for your physical well-being.

These need to be not only goals to shoot for, but MUST HAVES that will guarantee you better health, maintain your ideal weight, develop a stronger heart, stronger muscles, and guarantee that you will be in better physical shape in three months than you are now.

And unless you are eating healthy, forget about setting any kind of physical fitness goals. What you eat will account for at least 70% toward reaching your goals. Did you get that? Exercise all you want, but eat poorly and nothing will change!

I have a friend who for years went to the gym every other day. On the in between days, he either went swimming or running or biking. He set goals for losing weight, was working hard, sweating, burning calories and staying consistent 6 six days a week. The result? A stronger heart rate, but he could not lose any weight.

He finally hit the wall of frustration and decided he would also need to change his diet. He set goals for his eating plans and cut out the sugar, wheat and starchy carbs, and ate more plant-based foods. The result? He's 25 pounds lighter and buff.

You will have a much easier time getting in shape with profound physical changes if you combine your exercise routines with a solid nutritional plan.

So with that in mind, here are some basic guidelines you can use when setting your goals. I've gleaned much of this from Jack Canfield, a prolific author and life coach. He uses acronyms to describe them as **S M A R T** goals.

1. Specific.
Be clear and define your goal in simple terms. It should be precise, detailed and uncomplicated.

2. Measurable.
Without measuring you won't have a way to check your actual progress and ultimate outcome. And you can't measure without having specific targets.

3. Attainable.
Setting goals usually means you're looking to push yourself to or through a place that is beyond where you are. But you should be able to accomplish it within the constraints of your time, environment, abilities and resources.

4. Realistic.
Having a big breakthrough goal is good, but be realistic in achieving what you know is possible. So be realistic. Losing 100 pounds in 12 weeks won't happen if it is physically not possible.

5. Time Bounded.
Always set a target deadline for completion of your goal. Be specific with a literal time and date. "Lose 30 pounds in 12 weeks in order to weigh ____ pounds by 10:30 am on ____ (date)"

❑ **Write out your specific goals and include your food intake.**

Now comes the fun part. You've heard it before, "Fail to plan and you will plan to fail!"

4

Design Your Plan

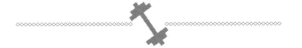

Start at the end point of your goal and break down what is needed by certain dates in order to hit your target.

Whatever your goal is, it's guaranteed you're not the first one to set that particular goal. That means there is help for you at the touch of your finger when you do an online search for what you're after.

So, whether it's losing fat and inches, gaining muscle, improving cardio, eating a healthy diet, improving your mindset or all of the above, someone has already designed a plan for you.

Years ago, a friend challenged me to run a 26.2 mile marathon. I was a casual runner and had never run further than three miles. So I set a goal to run the marathon on the specific date of the race and finish it in under four hours. After searching for "marathon training plans," I selected one that was 12 weeks long, using a day by day schedule of how far to run and at what pace.

It was a no brainer. All I had to do was follow the schedule and check it off each day, which I did. But I needed a strong why, and for me it was simply to do something I never thought I was capable of doing. So, I had a *why*, a *goal*, and a *plan*.

The result? I finished it and did it in 3 hours and 40 minutes. It was a huge confidence booster and something I look back on as a key stepping stone to other goals I achieved after that.

Now it would have been one thing to set this somewhat *out-there* goal, but without a detailed plan for how to achieve it, I would have failed. Sure, I may have thought to myself, I'm in relatively good shape so I'll just keep life as is, put the race date on my calendar, think about it for 12 weeks, and then just go out and run it. No plan, no training, no measurement benchmarks and no chance of finishing, guaranteed.

You get the idea. A good plan that breaks down the steps and the timeline is crucial in order to succeed.

So review your goals and then find a detailed plan that you will commit to follow through on until it's complete. If you search the internet or app store, you will find hundreds of thousands of fitness and nutrition plans, so it won't be hard to find exactly what you're looking for.

If you've never done this before, here are a few resources to check out as a starting point for you.

NUTRITION AND EATING

» **Films**. These documentaries will COMPLETELY alter your view of what you thought you knew about eating, dieting and nutrition.

Forks Over Knives (www.forksoverknives.com)
Plantpure Nation (www.plantpurenation.com)
What the Health (www.whatthehealthfilm.com)

» **The Daniel Plan** - www.danielplan.com
A highly successful plan based on the biblical Daniel's way of eating. Their site provides devotions, meal plans, small groups, videos, a fitness library, and it helps to get you started and keep you going.

» **Blue Zones** - www.meals.bluezones.com
This site is not only a great resource for healthy meals, but also gives reports on their ongoing research showing healthy lifestyles among the world's longest living people.

CARDIO

» **Michael Mosley's *The Truth About Exercise* documentary** – www.vimeo.com/51836895
This film will blow you away as it provides convincing, documented research that shows how short term, high intensity workouts of less than 10 minutes outperform 20-minute to 1-hour cardio workouts. (I switched to HIT training and it is far superior than long boring runs on a treadmill.)

STRENGTH TRAINING

» **Body Building** -
www.bodybuilding.com
This site has a wide selection of free workout programs that give daily workout routines with printable workout sheets, instructional videos on how to perform each exercise, and lots of articles to keep you motivated and well informed.

» **ATHLEAN-X with Jeff Cavalier** -
www.youtube.com/user/JDCav24
Jeff has loads of free content on his YouTube channel and is not only a great strength trainer, but a physical therapist who knows how the body functions in weight training or bodyweight exercise

» **Just Six Weeks App** -
www.itunes.apple.com/us/app/just-6-weeks/id580878681?mt=8

Want to do 100 push-ups, 20 pull-ups, 200 sit-ups, 150 dips and 200 squats? If you don't want to go to a gym or don't have any equipment at home, this is by far the best bodyweight fitness program you can find. This app offers five full-body exercises and lays out a six week daily routine based on your own progress to help you achieve each one of these goals. I've done it and it works! Check it out.

» **Get Visibly Fit in Mind, Body and Spirit** -
www.wendiepett.com

Wendie Pett, my wife, is a health and wellness coach and creator of the Visibly Fit program. You will find numerous resources on her site using a holistic approach to health and fitness.

A SAMPLE OF MY OWN HEALTH AND FITNESS REGIMEN.

Just by way of example and encouragement, let me give you a general overview of my own eating and workout routines. My quest for health and fitness didn't really kick in until I was in my late 40s. At the time of this writing I'm 68 years old and in better shape than I was almost 30 years ago. Consistency and self-discipline are the keys.

Because I've been doing this sort of thing for a while, I like to change things up quite often to stay motivated and prevent myself from falling into unproductive ruts. My goals and plans generally run along a six-week timeline. After I complete that round I typically take a week off and then begin a new program.

HOME GYM.

No gym memberships for me. My gym is in the basement and is super simple. I have a set of PowerBlock dumbbells that adjust from 10 pounds to 90 pounds each. Add to that an adjustable bench, and there is hardly an exercise routine I can't perform. In addition, I have some free weights and a rack if I want to get a bit more variety and heavier loads. I also have an adjustable chin up bar over my doorway, and a resistance band that I can use for just about any exercise.

When I travel, I often take along my resistance band that can attach over the door. Or I will do two to three sets of five exercise routines with bodyweight exercises (often using the Just Six Weeks App). Other times, I use a variety of my wife's *Visibly Fit* exercises found on her website.

STRENGTH TRAINING.

Workouts consist of three to four days in my home gym with either weights or bodyweight exercises, and two to three days of cardio/high intensity training. There is at least one day, and more often two days, of rest.

TRACKING.

I track everything by writing out what I do for each workout. I record the date, time, exercises, amount of weight used, reps, etc. I include anything that gives me a measurement of my progress so I can see how I'm doing compared with the last time.

CARDIO.

I hike or take accelerated walks with my wife or do ten minutes of high intensity that she designed. I call it the ten-minute torture! It's five exercises such as burpees, jumping jacks, fury squats, mountain climbers, and long jumps. You do one exercise all out for 30 seconds followed by a one to two-minute rest, and in ten minutes you are maxed out!

EATING PLAN.

For the most part, it stays pretty much the same from day to day. I'll eat five to six small meals a day. I have a very fast metabolism, so depending on how hard I'm training, I generally have to eat more than the average person.

My brother, Brad, taught me years ago to eat the Bible way. When I asked him what that was, he said, "If God grew it, you can eat it."

For occasional variety I will change up my eating routines, but in general, thanks to my wife Wendie, I eat a primarily plant-based diet consisting of any and all greens and vegetables, a few grains, and some rice and beans. However, I also add in Alaskan salmon and, on rare occasion, grass-fed beef and/or free-range chickens.

The small meals that I eat mid-morning and mid-afternoon are usually along the lines of a protein shake. Let me give you an awesome recipe for a great tasting protein drink that you can mix up in your blender. I call it the *Death Defying Shake*. Just add all of the ingredients to your blender and push the button. It's that easy.

DEATH DEFYING SHAKE (2 servings)
- 8 ounces of chocolate almond milk
- 1 large scoop (about 1 cup) plant-based protein powder
- 1 tablespoon of green drink powder of your choice (or handful of spinach)
- 1 cup frozen mixed berries
- 1 banana
- 1 teaspoon Udo's Oil
- 1 teaspoon almond butter
- 1 tablespoon apple cider vinegar
- 1 tablespoon cacao powder
- Sprinkle with ground cinnamon to taste
- Fill to top with water (6-8 ounces)
- Blend for 25 seconds

SUPPLEMENTS.

For years I've pretty much been a supplement junkie, experimenting with anything I thought might be lacking in my food. Unless you're eating completely organic (from a trusted, reliable source), it is hard to get the nutrients out of our chemical-saturated and depleted soil. However, I've now boiled it down to taking only what I believe are the essentials that I'm not getting enough from in the food I'm eating. I would recommend you consider these as well:

- CoQ10; B12; Magnesium Malate and Chelate; D3, Omega 3s; Ashwagandha, a probiotic and a variety of Green Powders.

That's pretty much my Health and Physical Fitness plan. Nothing complicated, but it does take intentionality and consistency. At this age, I've noticed that it takes longer to get back in shape if you lapse in any area. Whereas in your 20s and 30s, you have a much longer grace period.

There is one other very important key to help unlock your full potential in becoming fit and healthy.

Develop a *daily* routine.

It can be your secret ingredient to help you succeed in achieving your health and fitness goals. Having a routine is a discipline (helpful training) that will have huge payoffs in all areas of your life, and will keep you consistent. Here's a sample one that I like to follow to jumpstart my day.

- Wake up and thank God for another day and surrender everything to Him.
- Deep breathe five to ten breaths.
- Hang on a bar over the doorway to stretch out.
- Drink two large glasses of warm water with lemon juice, vinegar and red pepper.
- Spend time in devotions and prayer with a hot beverage, and most often with my wife.
- Make the bed.
- Do casual jumping on a rebounder for five minutes.
- Do ten minutes of various stretches for all body parts.
- Eat a bowl of oatmeal with berries, walnuts, coconut flakes and cinnamon.
- Shower and finish with a one minute cold rinse.
- Listen to a short podcast while finishing getting ready for the day.
- Start my work day!

This has become such a daily routine for me that when I travel and can't do all of it, it only makes me that much more grateful for when I can. The daily routine is not a chore. It's a pleasure and something that sets my day in motion in all the right ways.

Your daily routine can do the same. Whatever routine works best for you will make a difference, and empower you for the rest of your day.

MENTAL FITNESS

Before ending this section, let me mention something about spiritual and mental fitness. They are closely tied together. We covered the importance of spiritual fitness in Section 1 about quiet times. Practice this daily and you can almost guarantee mental fitness!

Why?

Because the more intentional time you spend pursuing God in prayer and reading His Word, the more your mind will be conformed to the same mind of Christ.

"Who has known mind of the Lord so as to instruct him? But we have the mind of Christ." 1 Corinthians 2:16 (NIV). When you read and study the Word of God, you are given spiritual insights that develop a supernatural mind – the mind of Christ.

"Do not conform to the pattern of this world, but be transformed by the renewing of your mind." Romans 12:2 (NIV).

As your mind is renewed, you will be able to better understand God's ways rather than simply conforming to the world's ways. Along with that, you are given the practical wisdom needed to know what to do in every area of life to bring honor to God and fulfill His purpose for you.

In addition, God has given us some incredible opportunities to develop our mind. And we can expand our base of knowledge on just about any subject matter you could conceive.

Anyone, just about anywhere in the world who has a computer or smartphone, has an entry point into any area of life you want to learn more about. From how to improve your job skills, to learning a new language, or anything else you can think of, there is an overabundance of content waiting for you.

A strong mind makes for a strong life, so be intentional in learning and developing your mind.

❒ Build a learning time into your daily routine. Spend time every day using podcasts, YouTube, audio books, articles, online classes, etc. It's all there for the taking.

Now, no matter how good your health and fitness plans are, or how well you practice these areas of fitness in mind, body and spirit, they will become worthless and you will fail unless you have someone, or a band of brothers, who can help hold you accountable.

You need someone who's got your back!

5

Stay Accountable

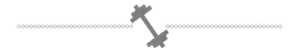

We've talked about this in the FAITH section under Don't Go It Alone. As you walk out your faith on a daily basis, staying closely connected and committed to a band of brothers, keeps you protected, encouraged and inspired.

This is equally true and important when it comes to your health and fitness. You need someone or a group of someones, to help you carry out your plans and reach your goals.

And of course with today's technology, there are incredible tools available that, when consistently used, can motivate you and give you data for measuring your results.

One of the absolute easiest and most painless ways to objectively stay accountable and track your health and fitness progress, is to use a simple Fitbit, Apple Watch or fitness app. My wife almost obsessively tracks her daily activity and competes against the pre-sets on her Apple Watch to reach her goals for steps, calories burned and exercise, before climbing into bed.

But while these are awesome tools and should be mandatory for anyone serious about getting fit, the truth is, they typically don't stay consistently in use.

Therefore, you really need to go the extra mile to guarantee yourself success. You need someone who will commit to help you out! It could be a trainer, a coach, a spouse or a true friend who is more fit than you. But you need a real human who you have to answer to and who will make the difference between you achieving your goals verses only *wishing* you could.

Maybe you want to get creative and use a whole bunch of humans to keep you accountable. If you're on social media, you already have hundreds of people watching you and tracking your story.

I saw an interview with a woman who wanted help losing a lot of weight after her pregnancy. So she posted her before pictures and stats on her Facebook page and asked her friends to help keep her accountable as she followed through on her weight-loss plan. She regularly posted pictures and videos of her steady progress.

Not only did she reach her target weight, but she went beyond and got in the best shape of her life. Today, she has an online health and fitness coaching business and is helping others do the same.

How is that for creatively keeping yourself accountable to work your plan and reach your goals?

My wife is a health and wellness specialist and naturopath. She coaches women one-on-one and in small groups. Her clients are typically looking to lose a lot of weight and get back their health. Almost every single one of them have tried multiple weight loss programs and diets, with little to no lasting results.

Why? There was no accountability.

But during my wife's seven-week Visibly Fit coaching program, there is daily accountability. Her clients have to report in every day with pictures of everything they eat, the exercises they perform, their weight, their measurements, even their mindset for that day. And they all commit to take it so seriously that if someone won't consistently follow through, she can fire them!

Now that's accountability.

So who's got your back in this area of your life? Unless you are incredibly self-disciplined, you're not going to make it on your own.

Check yourself on this. When was the last time you set goals and actually met them without any help from anyone? If you've got a good track record on this, congrats. Keep going and help others along the way.

But if that's not you, what will it take for you to make the changes this time around? Who will you go to and ask for help?

If it means hiring an experienced coach or trainer, do it. It will cost you. But it's an investment in you, and you will be more motivated to get your money's worth when you have to pay.

There is a scripture in the Bible that is often quoted during marriage ceremonies, but I think it applies in this area as well.

"Two people are better off than one, for they can help each other succeed. If one person falls, the other can reach out and help. But someone who falls alone is in real trouble" (Ecclesiastes 4:9-10).

Don't go it alone. Avoid the trouble and get someone to help you and hold you accountable.

❏ Take a few minutes to research fitness coaches, groups, Facebook communities and apps, and decide how you are going to be held accountable to your plan. Then make a commitment and put your start date on your calendar.

❏ **Check out our Facebook community for more ideas.**
FACEBOOK: What Every Man Needs to Know - faith, family, fitness, finances

MY COMMITMENT

Today's Date _____

I will be held accountable to _____

in the following way _____

_____

_____

_____.

I will begin on (date) _____.

Signature: _____

FINANCES

DICTIONARY.COM DEFINITION:

1. the management of revenues; the conduct or transaction of money matters generally...

2. the monetary resources, as of a government, company, organization, or individual; revenue.

FINANCES

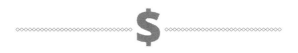

"Show me the money!"

That line out of the Tom Cruise movie, Jerry Maguire, pretty much tells the story for most American men. How much money you have is almost the badge of honor that proves your self-worth and validates your success.

But it's a lie.

We've been handed the wrong meaning of success. Check yourself out on that one. If you are asked to name a friend or acquaintance who is successful, it's likely you will identify someone who has above average income and material goods. It's the culture we grew up in and it's still prevalent today.

But you can change your mindset and live counter-culturally. Prove to yourself and others that money and possessions are not the standards by which your success will be measured. Jesus said, *"Life is not measured by how much you own"* (Luke 12:15).

Well, if how much I own is not the measure of success, what is? Best selling motivational author Stephen Covey once said, "If you carefully consider what you want to be said of you at your funeral, you will find your definition of success."

Do you have your definition of success?

As you think it through, you may want to use the Merriam-Webster definition as your starting point: Success is, "a favorable or desired outcome."

What do you want the outcome to be for your life?

Having lots of money, homes, cars, toys? Prestige, status, position? Or at the very minimum, a healthy 401k that allows you to live comfortably after you retire?

What's wrong with that? There is certainly nothing wrong, per se, with having retirement funds to live off and share with others. But if that is the outcome that determines your success, then you will be driven by the wrong motives and not succeed in the things that matter most.

❒ Take a moment right now and write out the definition of success for you. Record it in your journal or your notes app, but get it down and then memorize it. As you do, it will become part of you and help to retrain your brain.

Not only does it make a difference for you to redefine success, but it is equally important to get clear on your understanding of the meaning of money.

1

Understand the Meaning of Money

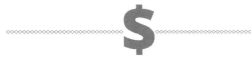

It's just a simple tool right?

Something generally accepted as a medium of exchange, a measure of value, or a means of payment in the form of coins and banknotes. In other words, it enables the owner to get what he wants if he has enough money to pay for it.

While that may be an objective, generalized meaning of money, most of us make it a subjective meaning, for personal interpretation and application.

The meaning of money and how it is used can be applied in multi-dimensional ways for different people.

For example money could be viewed as:

• Survival.
It pays for the basic necessities like food, clothing, shelter and transportation.

• Freedom.
Money allows us to do things we wish to do, from vacations to retirement.

- **Time.**

  It's been said, "time is money," but in reality, money is time. We trade our time for money and the money allows us to have more time.

- **Treasury.**

  When stored up, money can be a financially secure future for retirement and inheritances.

- **Status.**

  Having more money can mislead people into believing that riches define success and superiority.

- **Control.**

  Using money to master the circumstances of life can give a sense of security and power. (That idea is inherently false.)

- **Scorekeeper.**

  Money can be used as a metric to measure ourselves against others.

- **Means to an end.**

  The obvious outcome for using money is that it will achieve a particular end, from buying the basic necessities to being able to donate to a charity.

- **Evil.**

  Money can be seen as evil because of the negative impact it causes when misused.

Perhaps somewhere on this list is your understanding of the meaning of money or you may have something completely different in mind.

❐ Take another moment and write out your one or two sentence statement on the meaning of money for you.

For me, both the definition of success and understanding the meaning of money evolved over time. Had I been clear on it in my teens, likely I would have had a better relationship with money from the start, rather than always wishing I had more.

When I was an adolescent, one of my favorite TV shows was one called, *The Millionaire*. It was about an anonymous man who wrote one million dollar checks and had them delivered by his personal messenger to unsuspecting people. Each show taught a lesson about what can happen with such a large sum depending on how people use it. It was very revealing.

It was at that young age that I decided I wanted to be a millionaire and spoke about it often. I was so excited about what would happen if I could be handing out million dollar checks to people. However, as I got older, my motives changed and I didn't care as much about giving it to others as I did about making myself comfortable.

But as it turned out, after I surrendered my life to Jesus Christ, my perspective changed again. Money was no longer a driving force in my life. The spiritual eyes to see gave me the freedom to passionately pursue things that had more eternal payoffs.

I believed and practiced simple, biblical truths about money, and especially what Jesus taught about it. The end result is that, relatively speaking, I have more than I need and have been able to help others in need instead of self-indulging.

Once you get clear on your definition of success, apart from money, and understand the meaning of money, then you will be ready to manage it.

And it may seem obvious, but *the way in which you manage the money entrusted to you, will make or break how well most other areas of your life goes.*

But before diving into some basic rules for managing your money, we need to consider God's perspective and purposes for money.

2

Learn God's Take on Money

For those who believe that God has something to say about money, we can simply look to His Word and draw some pretty insightful conclusions.

The Bible offers 500 verses on prayer, fewer than 500 verses on faith, and more than 2,000 verses about money. In fact, 15 percent of everything Jesus ever taught was on the topic of money and possessions - more than His teachings on heaven and hell combined.

Now let's be honest. Just because there are more verses about money does not mean that it is a more important subject than things like prayer and faith. Instead, it just shows us how interwoven money is into our everyday lives.

Jesus warned us that you can't serve money and God. You will end up loving the one and hating the other. You will be devoted to the one and despise the other.

I take that to mean there is a huge temptation to distort the role money has in life. Once it becomes a preoccupation and takes priority in your life, it really becomes your master. (See Matthew 6:24.)

When that happens, you are at risk of losing your soul.

"What does it profit a man if he gains the whole world but forfeits his soul? Is anything worth more than your soul?" (Matthew 16:26).

Jesus also taught that wherever your treasure is, that's where your heart will be also. So if you spend yourself stockpiling your treasures here on earth, that will be the focus of your attention and you will lose it all in the end. You'll never see a hearse pulling a U-Haul because you can't take it with you!

❐ Stop for a moment. Be brutally honest with yourself. Where are you at with all this?

• Are you spending more of yourself on building wealth instead of nourishing your soul? Why or why not?

• Is making money the driving force in your life, and if so, what is the present outcome?

• Does money dominate too much of your time, thoughts and priorities, and if so, why?

• Have you stressed yourself out trying to accumulate treasures here on earth? Homes, cars, toys, retirement funds?

• Are you *serving* your money?

If you answered "yes" to any of these questions, don't read on until you make a decision to change something.

Commit to doing whatever it takes to turn things around so you don't have to stay stuck in the same place. In fact, you must not stay stuck, for the sake of your soul and for the sake of those you care about.

☐ Write out how you will change your answers from **yes** to **NO**.

•

•

•

•

☐ If you need to deepen your understanding of how crucial this is, take time to read more about what God has to show you about money. Check out Compass, a non-profit ministry that teaches people how to handle money based on the principles of the Bible.

This site, www.compass1.org/the-bible-on-money, will show you 31 different categories of how money affects you using 2,350 verses from the Bible.

If you want to serve God and not money, and be devoted to Him not to the demands of getting money, make every effort to follow His principles.

As I've spent years reading and studying God's principles on money, I've boiled them down to this very simple summary:

1. God owns everything.
2. Whatever I have in my possession is gifted by Him.
3. Since it is all His, I am to manage it for Him and His purposes.
4. Owe no man anything but the debt of love.
5. Storing up treasures on earth will do me no good in eternity.
6. Because I can't take it with me, investing in His work is the best way to lay up treasures in Heaven.

I pretty much use this as an overarching money management plan. It works for me, and in the next section I'll break out more of the specifics on how to effectively manage your money.

3

Manage Your Money

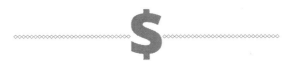

"He who is able to control his wallet will have the self-discipline to control every other area of his life!"

I made that up, but I believe it's true. Think about it. You have a relationship with money, and either it controls you, or you control it. Mastering the management of your finances will keep you free from a multitude of stressful problems that spill over into all other areas of life, from relationships to health.

Now, a word about men and money. As a man, I believe you have been given the primary responsibility to manage money in an exemplary way for those within your care.

One of the privileges of being a man is that you get to be a provider. But if you're busy providing and not managing the provision, you will fail. Too many times we see couples who end up in divorce because of problems with money, and often it is the man who didn't provide the leadership.

I have a married friend who didn't want to take the time or hassle of managing money. Of course his excuse was that he just wasn't good with money and they were better off with his wife handling all the finances. So she had to take the lead.

However, over time, problems developed with how and where the money was going. There wasn't open conversation about it, which led to multiple misunderstandings, and she grew resentful. She not only needed her husband's input, but his leadership. Thankfully, he is awakening to his role and they are now learning together how to manage their money.

I have another friend whose wife wanted him to manage the money and control where it went. He was a businessman and she assumed he knew a lot more than she did about money, and things would turn out better with him in charge. Unfortunately, he ran his household finances like he ran his business. He took risks, went into debt and spent more than he had. It brought the business and his household down. In hindsight, he learned that as a leader, he should have included her and they would have benefitted from her insight and intuition.

So as a man, take leadership with your finances whether you feel like it or not. Whether you think you're good at it or not. Don't abandon your responsibility. Balance things out by making certain to include your wife as part of your team effort, and run your finances in a way that will honor God and bless your family.

And remember, it truly is not complicated, but it does take knowledge, discernment and self-discipline. Just commit to following through and keep it simple.

John Wesley, the 18th century evangelist, kept it simple when teaching about handling money. "Make as much as you can, save as much as you can and give away as much as you can."

Nice huh? So how do we do that?

1. First and foremost, remind yourself daily that God owns it all.

Whatever you have within your possession is not really yours, but graciously on loan from the Owner. If you lose sight of that, you're on a slippery slope and nothing will line up with God's purposes for you and your money.

2. Take inventory.

Do a simple balance sheet of your assets (stuff of value you have that is free and clear of debt) and your liabilities (debts against the stuff you have). The difference between the two is your actual net worth (the total sum of how much money you actually have). As you evaluate your income, keep it in perspective. *"You shall remember the LORD your God, for it is he who gives you the power to get wealth"* (Deuteronomy 8:18).

3. Budget.

Here's a simple rule: never *let your outgo exceed your income*. Not knowing exactly how much you're spending against how much you're making usually ends up in financial disaster. Without knowing how much is going where, and whether you have enough to cover it, will put you in denial. Once in denial, you will compound your problems until at some point they will collapse in on you.

Whether you make a lot or a little, budgeting needs to be mandatory if you want freedom from financial stress. Putting together a budget is not difficult to do, and should be welcomed as one of the most helpful tools you can have for managing your money. There are multitudes of free, online resources and budget templates that can revolutionize your finances. Grab one, fill it out, and commit to living within your means.

4. Set Goals.

Along with budgeting is goal setting. "Aim at nothing and you will hit it every time." The benefit of setting financial goals, is that it creates both discipline and momentum. Keep God in the center of setting your financial goals and it can be a rewarding and exhilarating experience. Use the same basic format for setting financial goals as you did for your fitness goals.

☐ Get clear on exactly WHAT you want or need. (Be specific)

☐ Answer WHY you want or need that.

☐ Decide WHEN you want to achieve that goal.

☐ Design your plan.

I've used this process throughout my lifetime, including the years where my income was below the poverty line. But as I remained disciplined and faithful, setting goals based on God's principles, I was never lacking, and over the years, I prospered.

5. Get out of debt and stay out.

"Owe no man anything but the debt of love" (Romans 13:8). Can you imagine the freedom you experience when you don't owe anyone any money?

One of the best ways to avoid debt is to simply pay your bills on time and live within your means.

Don't use credit cards unless you can pay them off, on time, every month. You can save thousands of dollars annually if you avoid all interest charges.

Even though it can make sense to borrow for an appreciable item (like a house, not a car) there is no greater feeling than owing nothing. I had a very aggressive mortgage payoff plan and just recently sent in my last payment. No more debt gives tremendous freedom, joy and opportunity.

No matter how much debt you currently have, you can put an aggressive plan together that can get you completely debt free in less time than you think.

The best resource to go to is Financial Peace University by Dave Ramsey at www.daveramsey.com.

6. Save and Invest.

I lived by and taught my children what we called the 10-10-10 Rule.

- Give 10% of your income to God's work.

- Save 10% so that you can have at least 3 months cushion to pay for all your bills. After that, save for things you need to buy later, such as a car, vacations, education, appliances, etc.

- Invest 10%. This can be a complicated and risky area, so get professional help. Don't "play" the stock market. Use the rules of compounding and diversification. Don't invest any amount in anything with high risk unless you are willing to lose it all. Put your money primarily in those investments that help others. Remember, it's not yours, it's God's, so invest wisely as you manage it for Him.

7. Give to others.

Pastor and Bible teacher J. Vernon McGee once said, "Do your givin' while you're livin' so that your knowin' where it's goin'." As you journey along in life, there's great satisfaction in seeing how others can be impacted by your generosity as you share what God has entrusted to you. And amazingly, the more we give the more it seems to come back. Jesus said, *"Give and it shall be given to you, pressed down, shaken together and spilling over!"* (Luke 6:38).

Giving to others is not just something nice to do, it is required of you. In fact, the act of giving has already been wired into you by the greatest giver Himself. So check yourself out on this. Have you ever regretted being generous?

If you're a Christian, you've likely been taught that you should tithe or give away 10% of your income. While that should not be a legalistic rule, it could be at least a starting point.

R.G. LeTourneau, a businessman and inventor of earth moving machines, became a very wealthy man. As a Christian, he loved giving and decided to flip the 10% tithe percentage around. He committed to give 90% of his income and company profits to ministries and charities.

A friend of mine was making a very meager income when he first got married, but he loved to give. He constantly gave beyond his means, but the more he increased his giving, the more God provided for him and his growing family. *"You can't out-give God!"* was his constant declaration.

So, it's not a question of whether or not you should give, but rather, how much do you give and where do you give it?

Here is some simple criteria that I've used on how much and where to give:

• 10% of my before tax income is the starting place.
• Over and above that amount happens when I sense God giving me specific direction on something or someone in need.
• Outside of my immediate family, I give to any other extended family member in need.
• As God leads, I will give to friends, co-workers and sometimes strangers.
• God's Word shows His heart is for the widow (single moms, too), the poor, the sick, the imprisoned and those who are lost and need the gospel. So I give to ministries (including and especially my church) that specialize in those areas.
• If I'm uncertain about a non-profit organization, I first check their rating with a watchdog group like **Charity Navigator**, www.charitynavigator.org, or **ECFA (Evangelical Council for Financial Accountability)**, www.ecfa.org.

8. Pay your taxes.
While there is much wrong about the way in which our taxes are allocated, paying them is the right thing to do.

Jesus was asked about this by those who felt abused by Roman taxation and were trying to trip Him up with a trick question. But He settled the matter when He said: *"Give to Caesar what is his and to God what is God's"* (Mark 12:17).

Jesus proved he was willing to abide by this law and pay his taxes. Sure, He told Peter to go catch a fish and he would find the coin for taxes in the fish's mouth. (I wouldn't recommend trying that, but you never know.) The point is, that if even Jesus made good on His taxes, so should you.

Be smart in paying your fair share and don't cheat. In reality, there are certain benefits that come from paying taxes. Yes, the list seems shorter than the value you're getting, but seeing it with the right perspective will keep you free and joyful.

9. Commit to lifestyle changes.
Once you go through a process of becoming a good manager, or steward, of the finances God has entrusted to you, it will be almost impossible not to reevaluate your lifestyle. You will not only have a different perspective on money, you will have a better grip on what to do with it and why.

As you go through this process, you will become aware that money is just a tool. You will lose your attachment to it and its attachment to you. Freedom will follow. And if your lifestyle is too dependent on you making a lot of money, you will become more motivated to get free by simplifying your life.

Only you can answer how much is enough. But it becomes increasingly easier to want to accumulate less and give more when money is just a means, and not an end.

10. Get the Right Tools
Building your financial foundation is really not that difficult if you have the right tools. Too many times while working on some maintenance project around the house, I've heard myself say, "If only I had the right tool, this would be a lot easier."

Don't get me wrong. Having the right tools to work with is a big help, but it still takes a lot of work and self-discipline to consistently and correctly use those tools. Financial freedom does not just happen by itself. So again, before you put your master plan together, earnestly go through each of the previous points and keep strengthening your WHY for financial freedom.

There are endless websites, books, podcasts, online courses, in person classes and a long list of helpful resources dealing with your finances. Here are just a few, but reliable ones, that can be a good starting point for you.

» Role models.

Start here because it's true that "More is caught than taught." There are people around you whom God can use to show you how it's done. My mom was probably the best budget mentor alive. As a young boy I would watch over her shoulder as she explained what she had to spend money on and how she was going to do that with such limited income. I also modeled running my business by what I saw my dad do. He consistently used conservative but reliable business principles. Find your role model, your mentor, and ask for their help.

» Compass - finances God's way - www.compass1.org

Loaded with biblically-based, free resources for managing your finances.

» *The Treasure Principle* by Randy Alcorn.

This quick read will challenge you to rethink the meaning of money from the Bible's perspective.

» Dave Ramsey's Financial Peace University -
www.daveramsey.com

Everything you could ever want to know about managing money, getting out of debt, saving, investing, and giving. Ramsey has impeccable credentials and is a proven and trusted expert who has impacted countless numbers of people.

» Mr. Money Mustache - www.mrmoneymustache.com

Mr. Money Mustache is a fascinating character who is brilliant when it comes to a common sense approach to money. This site has resources to teach you how to simplify your life and gain financial freedom sooner than you think.

» *Unshakeable: Your Financial Freedom Playbook.*

This book by Tony Robbins is an abbreviated sequel to MONEY: Master the Game. It simplifies the complexities of managing and investing money by giving a step-by-step playbook to help you achieve your financial goals.

» A reputable fiduciary to manage your investment portfolio.

This is different than a brokerage house where commissions are made on your transactions. Fiduciaries are registered investment advisors (RIAs) who are required to put their clients' interests ahead of their own. They manage your investments for you, and it will cost you between .25% to 1% of your portfolio annually. But it is worth it if you have a substantial amount and don't want to do it on your own.

11. A Summary of Simple Rules for Managing Your Money.

Check off the ones you're already doing. For the ones you're still working on, set some goals, make-a-plan and follow through.

- ☐ God owns it all.
- ☐ You are His manager.
- ☐ Be the leader in managing finances in your family.
- ☐ Get the right tools.
- ☐ Take inventory of your current situation with your finances.
- ☐ Create a budget and stick with it.
- ☐ Pay your bills on time.
- ☐ Live within your means.
- ☐ Set financial goals.
- ☐ Get out of debt and stay out.
- ☐ Don't borrow unless it is for an appreciable asset (like a home).
- ☐ Don't lend money you're not willing to lose.
- ☐ Don't pay retail price. Buy only on sale or discounted.
- ☐ Use the "three-bid rule" when comparing pricing to get the best deal.
- ☐ Save at least 10% of your income.
- ☐ Invest.
- ☐ Don't invest any amount you're not willing to lose.
- ☐ Give generously.
- ☐ Pay your fair share of taxes.
- ☐ Commit to and simplify lifestyle changes.

A WORD ABOUT WORK AND CAREER

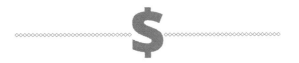

Undoubtedly, this is a subject that in and of itself, has many implications for the way in which it is tied into your everyday life. When it comes to finances, the work you do for the pay you get determines what you have to manage. Without work, there is no job or career. No job means no money, and no money means you can't provide for you or your family's basic needs. And honestly, it's about that simple.

So why is there so much attention on WHAT we do in life through our work? Shouldn't we first be more concerned with WHO we are in life? I'm guessing you'll agree, because who we are weighs more heavily in what we do and the way in which we do it.

Naturally, we want to believe that part of God's purpose for our lives here on earth is to fulfill His calling on our lives. But do we mistake His calling for the job or career we want or think He wants for us?

What if His calling is simply to know and love Him and be conformed into the image of Christ as His followers?

You may completely disagree with me on this, but I'm going to step out here a bit and say that your job is much less important than your calling. Your work is a means to an end. And to be sure, it is much more rewarding when your work is an expression of what you love to do and do well. Using your talents and skills in a job is not only fulfilling, but can bring tremendous honor to God who gifted you.

With that in mind, God gives incredible freedom for you to choose to use your talents and skills in whatever work you want to do in order to earn the income you need.

Should you seek God for guidance in your pursuit of work? Absolutely. But you also have His permission and blessing to pursue all the options out there. And as your loving Father, He certainly is able to lead you into the work you want to do.

So what if you're not yet able to do what you WANT to do, and instead are doing something you HAVE to do in order to have an income?

If you are an American, or live just about anywhere in the Western world, you are in a land of opportunity. So don't stop hunting for your right opportunity. Don't give up. Jesus said, *"Keep on asking and you will receive, keep on seeking and you will find, keep on knocking and the door will be opened to you"* (Matthew 7:7).

In the meantime, until that door opens, relax, trust God and *"Whatever you do, work at it with all your heart as working for the Lord rather than for people"* (Ephesians 3:23).

This is the attitude and behavior that should always govern anything we do for a job or career.

CONCLUSION

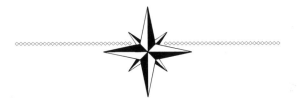

Unless you are living in solitude on a remote island or mountain top, these four areas of life – Faith, Family, Fitness and Finances – are woven together in your everyday existence.

You are, or will be, experiencing either success or failure, and joy or sorrow in some or all of these areas. It really depends on your choices. You have to own it and take responsibility for the outcome. There is no one else to blame if things don't go well. On the other hand, if the outcome is good, no one else made it happen for you either. You get the credit for all the hard work, the discipline, and the consistency in following through on a course of action that brings success.

Having said that, let me caution you to avoid stressing out over all of this and feeling overwhelmed.

Remember you already have what it takes.

God has given you His grace and power to carry out His purposes through you. He promised that He is the one Who began a good work in you and is faithful to bring it to completion. (Philippians 1:6)

Take the longer view of things and realize that it takes time to change things from the way they were to the way you want them to be.

Here is a suggestion that I want to encourage you to take to heart.

> Commit to a one-year timeline for making solid changes in these areas, so that you can give yourself the time and opportunity to succeed.

We have a beautiful potted palm tree that stopped growing. The only reason it stopped is because the pot was too small and the tree had no more room to enlarge itself. My wife repotted it so it now has the opportunity to reach its full potential. Even so, it won't happen overnight. But a year from now it will look magnificent.

You may feel like that palm tree, too confined in your present state and it's restricting your growth. All the more reason to replant yourself in the right environment. With a new state of mind and a solid plan of action, over time you will grow bigger on the inside and experience success in each one of these areas of life.

Prioritize each area and start with a concentrated effort in the one that needs the most help. You may want to spend three months on each one of these four areas as you set a one-year timeline. Go back through this guide and highlight the areas that are the most challenging. Reread certain sections and take note of what you underlined or highlighted, and take the time to develop an action plan. Check out the resources. Commit and immerse yourself until you prove to yourself that change can and is happening.

I have a grandson who needed to find out for himself what he was capable of in sales. He saved up and bought a world-class and expensive training course on how to master sales. He immersed himself in the training every day until he convinced himself he had what it takes. Within six months, he started setting record sales and became the company's number one salesperson.

Learning to master your faith, family, fitness and finances, guarantees that you will be much better equipped to fulfill your potential and carry out your role with purpose and satisfaction.

This is what men do.

They love a good fight, they love adventure in trying new things, and they love to compete against themselves to drive them to do and be better.

If nothing else, may what you just read throughout these chapters, at least stimulate your desire to want to grow and get better. Yes, it takes work and intentionality. It takes an effort to make changes, and seldom do changes happen without a certain measure of pain. But if you look at the outcomes in each area, your life will get better and you will have greater impact on those around you.

And while you will personally benefit, you already know that it's not really just all about you. It's about what happens to others around you when you are functioning at your peak and more fully-equipped.

That's living out your true purpose and calling – to honor God and love others.

And loving others can open up opportunities for you to help them, to serve them, and as a man, to fulfill your role to protect, provide and lead.

ABOUT THE AUTHOR

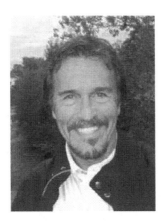

"You're never too old to learn something new and never too young to start learning a better way."

I know this to be true from my own experience. It's been a few years now since I've mined the depths of how to master these four crucial areas that impact our lives every single day.

Without a firm grip on your Faith, Family, Fitness and Finances, you will experience problems that cause hurt and pain for you and those around you.

I'm a guy and like you, I don't have much appreciation for being told what to do.

On the other hand, I have made enough mistakes to realize that until you learn, grow and master these four areas, you will likely keep repeating the same mistakes over. So, I'll never stop learning and growing and am hoping the same for you.

At age 29, I was fortunate enough to acquire a seminary education that gave me a much deeper dive into God's heart and a more insightful understanding of His word.

Any success I've experienced is the result of paying primary attention to the Biblical principles that govern these areas of life. That, and learning life hacks from experts and mentors in each one of the areas has given me a wealth of experience that has helped shape who I am and how I live my life.

As a former business owner of a media fundraising agency, I spent over 40 years consulting, training, coaching and encouraging media professionals. Today, I'm overlaying many of those principles in mentoring men who want to achieve success with their faith, family, fitness and finances. It's a journey worth taking so we can live out our purpose and fulfill our role as provider, protector and leader.

And along the way, I'll continue to cherish time with my wife Wendie as we travel and work together and enjoy our family gatherings with my two daughters, stepson and twelve grandchildren.

If you would like more information and a way to grow together you can find me here:

Facebook: What Every Man Needs to Know
www.facebook.com/groups/335136670551198/

Website: www.toddisberner.com
www.whateverymanneedstoknow.com

"If we really believe what we believe to be true,
how will we live our lives -
and if we don't live it out, do we really believe it?"

Made in the USA
Columbia, SC
22 February 2020

88287811R00085